The Vegetarian Sports Nutrition Guide

T0151371

The Vegetarian Sports Nutrition Guide

Peak Performance for Everyone from Beginners to Gold Medalists

LISA DORFMAN, M.S., R.D., L.M.H.C.

JOHN WILEY & SONS, INC.

New York   Chichester   Weinheim   Brisbane   Singapore   Toronto

The information contained in this book is not intended to serve as a replacement for professional medical advice. Any use of the information in this book is at the reader's discretion. The author and the publisher specifically disclaim any and all liability arising directly or indirectly from the use or application of any information contained in this book. A health care professional should be consulted regarding your specific situation.

Library of Congress Cataloging-in-Publication Data:
Dorfman, Lisa
    The vegetarian sports nutrition guide: peak performance for
    everyone from beginners to gold medalists / Lisa Dorfman.
        p.   cm.
    Includes bibliographical references and index
    ISBN 0-471-34808-2 (pbk.)
    1. Athletes—Nutrition.   I. Title.
TX361.A8D67   1999
613.2'024'796—dc21   99–25294

Printed in the United States of America
10 9 8 7 6 5

To my husband, Bob,
the "Wind Beneath My Wings"

Contents

▶ Part One Food as Fuel

Foreword

THE HUMAN BODY is the simplest yet most complex bit of working machinery. It is a marvel of movement, engineering, grace, and strength in sport with, possibly, a "million-mile motor"—if given the right fuels. Each new day provides new knowledge and usable information about fueling this magnificent machine to maximize fitness and performance.

In *The Vegetarian Sports Nutrition Guide,* Lisa Dorfman scores by giving 10- to 100-year-olds ways to maximize optimal fitness. Matching vegetarian nutrition to exercise makes this book an operator's manual that will have a lasting positive impact on quality of life for many who might have become couch potatoes with bad bodies.

Eating and exercise do not take vast amounts of time, and both can become enjoyable within the limits of progressive moderation. Exercise programs or diet plans are merely outlines, so remember, too much may lead to failure; a little bit can lead to more and more success. If you grasp Lisa's concepts of progression, apply them, and selectively modify them, you are well on the way toward winning performance and personal satisfaction that will give you a high quality of life as you move down the road. Keep in mind that you can have a changed energy system with the guiding principles that Lisa provides in this nutrition text, which has a basis of sound science and experience tied onto it.

It may not be outlandish to believe that "when you feel good, you have more energy, you move quicker, and you just feel better about yourself." If that is not a winning combination of factors that can generate a healthy America, one has yet to be discovered. Lisa Dorfman has created vast opportunities for everyone.

Bob Beeten
Director, Sports Medicine
United States Olympic Committee

Preface

SPORTS AND EXERCISE have been a major part of my life ever since I can remember. As a child I was always on the go. I didn't walk to school, I ran. Neighborhood boys asked me to join their pickup games. Later, I became something of a female "jockette," excelling in cross-country, track and field, baseball, and basketball. And since then, I have enjoyed a good deal of success as a professional marathon runner and triathlete.

Many say my achievements can be chalked up to genetics, along with a dose of hard work and determination. I won't deny that I am blessed in many ways, but I believe that 98% of my speed, strength, and endurance is due to one thing—my diet.

For more than two decades, I have been a vegetarian. It all started at the age of 15 when my Austrian-born mother returned to the workforce and my 50-year-old father retired and became "Mr. Mom." My life would never be the same.

Despite my dad's faith, genetics, and athletic background, occupational stresses had taken the best years of his life. His health concerns were mounting. High cholesterol, high triglycerides, high blood pressure, and diabetes were just the beginning.

Dad's days of meat, potatoes, beer, and ice cream obviously weren't working for him as he entered midlife. But then he read about Nathan Pritikin, the vegetarian guru of the 1970s. Dad became convinced that he needed to adopt a 10%-maximum-fat/vegetarian diet plus an exercise program to get his life and health back in control. It was a last resort before trying prescription drugs and psychotherapy.

I was shocked to see a grown man give up his meat and potatoes. But he did. And every day he prepared a menu of vegetables, grains, fruits, and plenty of supplements. He also started bicycling 20 miles a day. I supported his effort by giving up my preteen diet of fast food burgers, french fries, Diet Coke, and ice cream. Dad lost weight and reduced his levels of cholesterol, triglycerides, and blood sugar and pressure. He achieved—and maintained—15% body fat while thriving on a vegetarian diet that allows fish (pesco-vegetarian). For me, Dad's change laid the groundwork for my future as a nutritionist, psychotherapist, and coach.

I've never looked back since giving up chicken, fish, and red meat. In 1992, Hurricane Andrew destroyed Miami and my life. Our possessions blew as far as the Bahamas. Yet later that year I ran the best major marathon I had ever run, beating my personal record by 10 minutes and placing second overall at the Olympic Marathon course in Atlanta. Six months after giving birth to my third child, breastfeeding, and dealing with the stress of new motherhood again, I finished my first half-ironman—five hours of ocean swimming (1.2 miles), bicycling (56 miles), and running (13.1 miles). Since 1990, I have won or placed in the top 1 or 2% in 18 marathons, a 50-kilometer road race, and hundreds of triathlons, duathlons, and 5K to 30K road races. I've competed from sea level to 14,000 feet altitude and from 16°F to 100° F.

Why This Book?

For several years now, I have taught athletes at every level and every age how to enhance their performance with food. A good many of the athletes have been vegetarians at some time in their lives, but many more were not.

When I set out to write *The Vegetarian Sports Nutrition Guide,* I knew it would interest two types of people: affirmed vegetarians who know or suspect that they are not getting the most from their diet, and nonvegetarians who may or may not be curious about eating more of a plant-based diet but are definitely looking for an edge in their sport. Which describes you?

Eating a vegetarian or plant-based diet won't automatically elevate you to the top ranks of your sport or activity. If you're a weekend athlete, a vegetarian diet won't suddenly allow you to bicycle or jog twice your normal distance. Nevertheless, a well-chosen vegetarian diet will help you feel stronger and healthier. Just ask the 17 top vegetarian athletes who contributed their insights to this book.

For Dave Scott, six-time ironman champion, being a vegetarian athlete means "never having ups or downs in training performance and having the ability to refuel easily afterward." For Art Still, a six-foot-seven-inch, 255-pound former Kansas City Chiefs football player, a vegetarian diet helped build energy and endurance and decrease body fat. Other athletes such as Ben Williamson, a world-class sailor, and Debbie Stephens, a world-class equestrian show jumper, find that being a vegetarian helps them stay at their best competitive weights.

The benefits of a vegetarian diet rich in complex carbohydrates, fiber, and naturally low-fat foods are well known and numerous. But science is just discovering the magic of the micronutrients and compounds that exist in plant-based foods. These ingredients help maximize the potential energy available in the muscles and protect important cells in our bodies.

The Vegetarian Sports Nutrition Guide shows you how to maximize the benefits of a vegetarian diet for your specific athletic needs. Though you're welcome to read it cover to cover, feel free to skip around. In 10 chapters, you'll find juicy, hands-on sports nutrition advice. Part One explores food's impact on physical activity and sports, including the best "fuels" for your body—from the macronutrients (carbohydrates, protein, and fats) to the micronutrients (vitamins, minerals, and phytochemicals). In Part Two, you'll discover specific ways to use a vegetarian diet to reach your athletic goals.

If you are not a vegetarian and perhaps even a bit apprehensive about switching to a plant-based diet, you will learn how to adapt simple formulas, recipes, and tips to enhance your nutritional health as well as your training and fitness program. If you've already made the switch to a vegetarian diet, you will learn new and easy ways to reenergize your current eating regimen from the pros. Regardless of your activity level, you will have a better understanding of sports nutrition science and get a behind-the-scenes look into the lives of world-class vegetarian athletes.

The athletes profiled in this book were not raised vegetarian. They elected to make the switch in their teens or adulthood while pursuing more serious, high-level training and competition. They represent a variety of ages, sports, and cultural backgrounds. They also follow different types of vegetarian eating programs, from semivegetarian to lacto-ovo vegetarian to vegan. Their inspiring stories reflect how a plant-based diet can be applied to any sport at any level.

The goals in this book have broad applications and scientific support, also. They comply with federal dietary guidelines and the United States Department of Agriculture's Food Guide Pyramid. They also meet the recommendations of other recognized pyramids such as the Mediterranean and Asian pyramids, which are plant-based, and the American Heart Association and American Cancer Society guidelines.

While these guidelines have slightly different takes on what it means to eat healthfully, they all validate the need for a diet rich in carbohydrate fuel, stabilized with protein and sprinkled with fat, glued together with a variety of vitamins, minerals, herbs, and phytochemicals. In *The Vegetarian Sports Nutrition Guide,* I apply these guidelines to the needs of active individuals like you by providing

► energy, carbohydrate, protein, and fat "formulas"

► fluid, vitamin, and mineral recommendations

► plant-based menus for peak performance

One of my goals for this book is to take sports nutrition beyond simply eating specific foods for a purpose. A vegetarian diet is rich in tastes and textures. And contrary to popular belief, vegetarians are more than just granola-eating former hippies or picky eaters who pore over food labels checking for meat and animal byproducts. Recent research from The Women Physicians Health Study suggests that 69% of female physicians who describe themselves as vegetarians do so for health reasons. Also, surveys of consumers from health food stores, traditional supermarkets, and a vegetarian food fair from 1974, 1992, and 1997, respectively, cited health consistently as the major impetus for a plant-based diet.

Vegetarians are passionate people who believe in themselves, their faith, the earth, and our children's future. They also savor good food. That's why I enlisted spa chef Jason Hanners, a former student of mine at Johnson and Wales University, to create simple, fast, and tasty recipes for vegetarian appetizers, soups, salads, main courses, and desserts. Jason experienced his own "plant-based conversion" when he adopted a semivegetarian program 2 years ago and lost 115 pounds.

I'd like to share three important points before you read further:

1. The food companies and products mentioned in *The Vegetarian Sports Nutrition Guide* have not provided any financial support in exchange for appearing in the book. They were selected based on recommendations from the athletes, Chef Hanners, or myself.

2. The recipes throughout the book have been placed in chapters or sections that relate to the composition, ingredients, or nutrient density of the food. Sometimes they just pop up, so don't be surprised!

3. Whenever you change your normal diet, activity, or lifestyle habits, ask your primary health care provider, such as your physician, if the program is suitable for your age and medical status. Do not attempt any program before getting the go-ahead from the medical professional who knows your needs best.

After completing the book, continue your transformation to a peak performance, plant-based diet by contacting me at my Web site (www.lisadorfman.com) for additional guidance and assistance.

Giving Back

In an effort to give back to the future and create great American athletes, I took a great deal of time and effort before starting this book to select a nonprofit organization that could benefit from a portion of the income that I receive from this book. I selected the SportsMed 2000 Program of the United States Olympic Committee (USOC).

SportsMed 2000 is a sports medicine program formed by the USOC to raise funds for education, research, program development, and equipment that is not available within the current USOC budget. The funds will ensure the best health care systems, education programs, research methods, medical technology, and nutritional guidance to help each athlete achieve his or her goals.

According to Bob Beeten, USOC Sports Medicine Director, the program "ensures the best possible sports medicine care for U.S. athletes in a cutting edge environment, and serves as a resource center for the dissemination of information for the entire Olympic sports community."

I made a commitment to give 10% of my net proceeds from this book to SportsMed 2000 to support America's athletes in 2000 and beyond. This is my way of passionately giving back to the sport and profession that I love.

Forever healthy, fit, fast, and vegetarian . . .

Lisa

Acknowledgments

I am grateful to the Lord God, who walks me through every challenge and success in my life.

To my children, Rebecca, Danielle, and Joseph, who reflect His miracles and love and my "vegetarian pregnancy diet" every day in every way.

To my mother, Melanie, who taught me to be strong regardless of life's circumstances, and my father, Walter, who encouraged me to be a vegetarian when I was 15.

To my siblings, Bruce and Linda, for being my role models in love and life.

To the athletes spotlighted in this book, who lent their time and talents and shared their strength, beauty, and passion for their vegetarian lifestyles.

To my dear friends, training partners, and colleagues who have molded me into the person, athlete, nutritionist, and mom I had always dreamt of being.

To mystery author James W. Hall, my neighbor and friend, who inspired me to write from my mind, heart, and soul.

To former *Miami Herald* sports reporter David Kilmer, my editor and friend, for his faith, honesty, and guidance.

To Gloria Mazer, L.M.T., my massage therapist since 1992, who has helped me to stay physically and mentally fit between competitions and the "chapters" of my life.

To Barbara Barbier, B.S.F. Teaching Leader, and my B.S.F. sisters for their fellowship, love, and support.

Introduction

FOR MANY PEOPLE, especially Americans, no meal is complete without meat. It is a tradition. Nonetheless, it is a relatively young tradition.

The earliest example of a plant-based diet dates to about 400,000 to 360,000 B.C. in the middle of the Pleistocene period, during which man "used fire to cook venison which supplements his diet of wild plants (hackberry), roots, nuts, acorns, legumes, and wild grains." God even inspired vegetarianism into the writing of the Old and New Testaments, beginning with the book of Genesis: "Everything that has a breath of life in it I will give every green plant for food" (Genesis 1:30).

Historically, most of the world has eaten a largely vegetarian diet. Only in affluent areas such as Europe and North America, where most citizens could afford meat and meat products, has a diet centered around meat become traditional.

In the United States, vegetarian diets didn't get much attention until the 19th century. Sylvester Graham, a Presbyterian clergyman and author, publicly attacked meats, fats, white bread, and even mustard, ketchup, and pepper, calling these foods "injurious to the health and stimulating to carnal appetites." Graham's popular book, *A Treatise on Bread and Breadmaking,* and his vegetarian-based hotel chain brought vegetarianism to the masses as thousands flocked to consume vegetarian diets. The champion of the vegetarian movement came in

1876, when the Seventh Day Adventist and surgeon John Harvey Kellogg created vegetarian foods and fed them to thousands who visited his Michigan retreat. He noted, "How can you eat anything that looks out of its eyes?"

The relationship between vegetarian diets and sports performance was first recognized in the 1800s. Initially, a preeminent physiological chemist promoted the concept that protein was the sole fuel source for all muscular movement. Research in the 1850s proved this theory false. Indeed, carbohydrates and fats were found to be the major sources of fuel for muscles.

Vegetarian athletes of the mid- to late 1800s were some of the first to prove the superiority of a plant-based diet, especially in endurance events. The London Vegetarian Society formed an athletic and cycling club that outperformed meat-eating competitors. Vegetarian athletes dominated walking races. In a German 100-kilometer walk, 11 of the top 14 finishers were vegetarians. In 1912, the vegetarian runner Kolehmainen became one of the first men to finish a marathon in under two and a half hours. Numerous other achievements and studies from this period reinforced the success of vegetarian diets for sport.

Recently, a California scientific researcher compared 351 vegetarians to 8,891 omnivorous runners and revealed that vegetarian runners average 13 to 14% more miles per week than non-vegetarians, have slimmer waists and lower total and LDL cholesterol by 3 to 5% (see chapter 5), and drink less alcohol.

Vegetarians of All Types

There are many different types of vegetarianism. There is even a distinction between a vegetarian diet and a plant-based diet. According to the American Institute on Cancer Research, a plant-based diet is more than eating garden flowers. A plant-based diet is "scientific lingo for a diet that consists primarily of vegetables, fruits, grains, and other foods from plant sources. It's different than a vegetarian diet in that it may include modest amounts of meat with an abundance of vegetables and fruits."

Vegetarian diets, on the other hand, eliminate animal products to different degrees.

▶ Types of Vegetarian Diets ◀

Semivegetarian	Includes some but not all groups of animal-derived products, such as meat, poultry, fish, seafood, eggs, milk, and milk products
Lacto-vegetarian	Includes milk and milk products but excludes eggs, fish, seafood, and meat
Lacto-ovo-vegetarian	Includes only milk, milk products, and eggs
Ovo-vegetarian	Includes only eggs
Vegan	Excludes all animal products, including eggs, milk, and foods that include animal byproducts
Fruitarian	Eats only fruits, nuts, honey, and olive oil
Macrobiotic vegetarian	Restricts animal products and progresses to a specific regimen "balance" of grains, fruits, vegetables, and some fish using in part the yin/yang philosophy and following a specific lifestyle that includes meditation, washing rituals, and special food preparation

A Healthy Kick

The health benefits of vegetarianism are numerous, according to clinical and experimental research studies as well as a position statement issued in 1998 by the American Dietetic Association.

One major advantage to consuming a plant-based diet is the reversal of coronary heart disease, shown most recently by Dean Ornish, M.D., and his Preventive Medicine Research Institute. His program demonstrated that arteries that have become clogged with fatty deposits actually respond to lifestyle and dietary changes, including a low-fat vegetarian diet, stress management, smoking cessation, moderate exercise, and emotional support. Mortality from coronary heart disease is lower in vegetarians. This appears to be due to the diet's naturally low content of fat, saturated fat, cholesterol, and animal protein. The typical vegetarian diet, compared with a meat-based diet, also has more folate (which reduces levels of homocysteine, thus reducing the risk for coronary heart disease), antioxidants such as vitamins E and C, and carotenoids (vitamin A), as well as phytochemicals.

Other health benefits of a vegetarian diet include reduced rates of hypertension, perhaps due to higher potassium intake; a lower incidence of death from Type 2 diabetes due to a higher intake of complex carbohydrates; less obesity; and lower body mass indexes (BMI). Constipation and diverticulosis are also less common in people who consume a high-fiber vegetarian diet.

Reduced rates of lung and colorectal cancer have also been shown, likely because of the abundance of dietary fiber, vegetables, and fruits consumed. Lower estrogen levels in vegetarian women may also protect against breast cancer. A 1998 study published in the *American Dietetic Association Journal* reported less oxidative DNA damage and lower breast cancer risk when consuming cooked vegetables versus a diet with meat.

A vegetarian diet may also treat or prevent conditions such as renal disease, osteoporosis, and portal-systemic encephalopathy (a disease of the brain). A low incidence of kidney stones has also been found in vegetarians. Some plant proteins decrease proteinuria (excess protein in the urine) and improve other kidney functions such as glomerular filtration rate and renal blood flow.

Vegetarians seem to absorb and retain more calcium from food. Lacto-ovo-vegetarians, for instance, have been shown to have the same calcium intakes as nonvegetarians. However, the lower protein intakes of vegetarians causes a calcium-sparing effect (see chapter 7). In addition to regular weight-bearing exercise and a low sodium intake, this may help prevent osteoporosis in susceptible women.

Environmental Concerns

Besides the health benefits offered by a vegetarian diet, there are also environmental implications. Modern methods of animal production waste energy and deplete topsoil. The grain used to feed animals provides only a fraction of the energy involved in eating the grain. For every 100 calories of plant material eaten by a cow, only 10 calories are stored in the cow, and one pound of pork provides 1,000 to 2,000 calories yet requires 14,000 calories to produce. It takes an average of 430 gallons of water to produce one pound of meat. And more vegetarians means fewer animals raised specifically for human consumption.

Waste materials associated with animal production are also a concern. Manure from overcrowded areas pollutes rivers and lakes. Excess nutrients cause algae growth that chokes aquatic life and causes nitrate pollution of drinking water. Animal waste produces gases that are released into the atmosphere, contributing to acid rain. Forests are also being cleared for new grazing land, diminishing the earth's ability to absorb carbon dioxide. This, along with the methane produced by animal waste, may contribute to global warming.

In the end, a plant-based diet is not only beneficial for the health of individuals, athletes, and families, it is important for the future of our planet.

▼

Food as Fuel

1

The Plant-Based Sports Engine

A T AGE 64, RUTH HEIDRICH should be an inspiration to us all. After being diagnosed with breast cancer in 1982, Ruth participated in a research project with Dr. John McDougall, a pioneer in the use of nutrition as medicine, and transformed her diet and exercise program. Ever since, Ruth has found no challenges with being a vegan, completely animal-free. In fact, she says it gives her more endurance and speedier recoveries from the six ironmans and over 700 road races, triathlons, and marathons she has completed.

In 1997 alone, Ruth completed 63 races, including the Senior Olympics. She's run the Great Wall of China, the Ironman New Zealand and the Ironman Japan (placing first in her age group), the Moscow Marathon, and other races all over the world. In her "spare" time at home in Hawaii, she hosts her own radio show, *Nutrition and You,* and has written two books, *A Race for Life: From Cancer to Ironman* and *The Race for Life Cookbook.* She has also given over one hundred talks every year since 1988.

Ruth takes no medications, alcohol, or even supplements. Her daily diet includes oatmeal, greens, Ruth's Ironwoman Pho (Vietnamese soup, which is her favorite one-pot meal; see page 149 for the recipe), brown rice, vegetables, baked potatoes, carrots, popcorn, and apples. Her favorite prerace meal is a special blend of brown rice, kale, banana, and blackstrap molasses (see page 37). Her favorite snacks include air-popped popcorn, sweet potatoes, apples, and carrot sticks.

I chose Ruth as the first vegetarian athlete to spotlight in *The Vegetarian Sports Nutrition Guide* because she inspires even the best athletes in the world and anyone else with an appreciation for the energy one needs to fight and overcome disease, let alone begin an admirable sports career at the age of 41. To me, Ruth represents the ultimate plant-based sports machine.

So, how does Ruth make the best use of carbohydrates, fats, and proteins in her vegan diet? How does she convert the energy from food to fuel her body for training, sport, and life? How does her vegan, plant-based eating program enhance her body's ability to compete at peak performance and recover quickly for everyday tasks?

Let's begin to tackle these questions by learning how the body uses and translates the nutrients from food to energy.

Warmup Session

Get ready for a condensed version of Energy Metabolism 101. I have tried to simplify some complicated terminology, but like cars, some of the words are not "convertible." After you read this section, you'll have a better appreciation for the impact and necessity of a plant-based diet for peak sport performance.

Picture your body in continuous motion—from bed to shower, work or school to sport, meals to reading, TV to sleep. To support these activities, the body is in constant need of energy, or calories. In addition to fueling the muscles to contract and relax for exercise, calories are used for

> ▶ digestion, absorption, and assimilation of food

> ▶ glands such as the pancreas and thyroid to secrete hormones like insulin and thyroxin, which help your body to function at rest and during exercise

> ▶ proper electrochemical messages from the brain to pass through nerves and stimulate muscles to contract and relax

> ▶ the synthesis of new compounds, such as protein for building larger muscle tissue through strength training

Though calories are found in carbohydrates, proteins, and fats, the body cannot unlock energy directly from these nutrients. Instead, the immediate source of energy is a chemical found in all cells, adenosine triphosphate (ATP). ATP is composed of a molecule of adenine and the sugar molecule ribose bonded with three phosphates, each consisting of phosphorus and oxygen atoms. When the outermost bond to the last phosphate is broken, it releases a tremendous amount of energy, so much energy that Johns Hopkins University researchers call ATP "one of the tiniest and most powerful motors ever identified."

ATP energy enables an athlete like Mark McGwire to hit his next home run, Wayne Gretzky to hit his last winning hockey goal, and Lance Armstrong to sprint for the finish of his Tour de France victory.

Only three ounces of ATP can be stored in the body at one time, which allows only a very short period of 0 to 4 seconds of high-intensity exercise. Fortunately, the supply of ATP can be rebuilt.

The ATP Energy Roadmap

Your body has two major energy systems that stimulate the transformation of ATP to fuel exercise: anaerobic and aerobic metabolism.

System 1a: The Power System

> Primary fuel: high-energy phosphate bonds of ATP and creatine phosphate (CP)
>
> Examples of sports fueled: heavy weightlifting, field events in track and field, and vaulting in gymnastics

The power system is the first one to kick in when energy is needed immediately. It feeds off ATP and creatine phosphate (CP), which supplies the "backup" phosphate needed for ATP to release its energy. CP has five times more energy than ATP and is "on call" 24 hours, but it is also in short supply. The body's specialized use of CP is the reason some athletes take and may benefit from creatine supplements to "juice up" these limited energy stores. Several athletes profiled in this book use creatine as a sports supplement. (See chapter 8 for information on creatine supplementation for short-term power exercise.)

The ATP–CP team is why we can produce a tremendous burst of

strength or speed—in football, tennis, track and field, golf, volleyball, karate, baseball, weightlifting, you name it—without taking a breath. In this anaerobic environment, and as activity continues for several seconds, carbohydrates are the only nutrient that can provide energy for the formation of ATP through glycolysis. Hence, high-intensity exercise relies on carbohydrates for energy.

System 1b: The Speed System—Anaerobic Glycolysis

Primary fuel: glucose (sugar)

Examples of sports fueled: running 200–800 meters, swimming 50–100 meters

If the demand for energy persists longer than a few seconds to a minute, ATP and CP stores become depleted. With specific enzymes, though, glucose in muscles can break down to another compound called pyruvic acid to produce new molecules of ATP.

Even so, this energy system, which is anaerobic because it doesn't require oxygen, supplies only a small amount of ATP. Large amounts of ATP needed to sustain a prolonged effort can only be generated by providing the muscle with more nutrients and oxygen. That's where the body's next energy system kicks in.

System 2: The Endurance System—Aerobic Metabolism

Primary fuels: carbohydrates, fats, and protein

Examples of sports fueled: marathons, long-distance swims, century bike rides, ironman triathlons, and other continuous events such as cross-country skiing

Although most energy is derived from anaerobic metabolism at the initiation of exercise, as activity continues the proportion of energy derived from aerobic metabolism increases. In fact, with oxygen, about 50 times more ATP can be made from stored muscle glycogen than with the two anaerobic systems combined.

Aerobic metabolism works by using hydrogen donated from fats and protein as well as acetyl Co-A, which is converted from pyruvic acid. Acetyl Co-A has a passport to the cell's powerhouse—the mitochondria, where more than 90% of ATP is produced. In this system, two vitamin B–containing enzymes called flavin adenine dinucleotide

(FAD) and nicotinamide-adenine dinucleotide (NAD) are required to direct the production of ATP. This process is also known as the Krebs cycle, named after the chemist who won the Nobel Prize in 1953 for this discovery.

Knowing that ATP is the primary source of muscle energy can and should impact how you exercise and eat. This is true whether your goal is to improve your general fitness or reach a new competitive level. The key is improving your ability to generate ATP.

Muscle Sense

Now that you understand how energy is generated for your power, strength, and endurance, you can find out how your muscles play a role in how you use ATP energy.

Genes largely determine muscles. We all have a genetic code for specific types and distribution of muscle fiber in all parts of our bodies. These individual muscle differences are responsible for producing elite marathon runners, sprinters, and gymnasts.

There are two types of muscle fibers:

1. White or fast-twitch fiber.   This class of muscle cells is best able to contract anaerobically. These so-called sprinter's muscles work twice as fast as slow-twitch fibers, depend almost entirely on anaerobic fuel for energy, and work great for short-term sprints and all-out efforts. Fast-twitch fibers, when exercised, will increase in size and in their ability to generate ATP. The overall result will be a bigger and stronger muscle. You know you have predominately these types of muscles if your specialty is power, strength, and speed.

2. Red or slow-twitch fiber.   These fibers are best able to provide ATP from oxygen and nutrients; in other words, to contract aerobically. The best endurance athletes in the world have these "marathon muscles." People with well-developed slow-twitch fibers are more energy-efficient and can train long hours because their muscles have more mitochondria (the metabolic portion of the cell) with more oxygen and enzymes for aerobic metabolism. Slow-twitch fibers, when exercised, will increase their capacity to produce ATP without increasing

in size. Many of the athletes in this book, such as Ruth, Dave, Ben, Jane, Gary, Jonathan, and myself, are "slow-twitchers."

Think of your body as having an ice cream parlor of muscle flavors. Although the flavors never change, they can be mixed to create new ones. In other words, even though we are born with a specific muscle fiber code, training can improve the flavor of muscles we possess.

The chart on page 15 shows the energy systems used for a variety of activities. You can cross-train with other sports or activities to improve your weaker energy system and muscle groups for your favorite sport. For instance, if you are great at sprint sports, or the Power and Speed system, and want to improve your aerobic system, endurance training can increase the amount of blood the heart pumps every minute to supply more oxygen to exercising muscle, which allows you to use more aerobic fuel or food energy, and can increase the mitochondria content in muscle, which increases the quantity of enzymes to use more food fuel, especially fat.

Fueling the Machine

Exercise and training improve the efficiency of the body's energy systems. However, you still need to fuel the machine.

As research and the athletes in this book demonstrate, a vegetarian diet can be the body's best fuel—with ideal proportions of carbohydrates, proteins, fats, and many of the vitamins and minerals necessary for sports and daily fitness activities. No, it's not as easy as swearing off meat and eating only vegetables. Peak performance requires effort and knowledge, no matter what the endeavor. For vegetarian athletes that means ensuring an intake of nutrient-dense plant-based foods critical to sports performance.

Caloric Needs of Vegetarians

There has been little information published regarding the actual dietary intake and eating behaviors of athletes. One study in 1984 examined the wide range of caloric intakes of athletes. In general, the size of the athlete and demands of his or her sport influenced the number of calories consumed each day. In this study, female dancers consumed as little as 900 calories per day and football players consumed the highest amount (11,000 per day).

▶ Major Sports and Their Predominant Energy Systems ◀

If you excel in power sports that are 50% or more fueled by ATP and CP, such as

Track and Field: 100–200
   meters, field events
Volleyball: beach and court
Figure skating
Bodybuilding
Equestrian
Karate
Skiing: downhill
Powerlifting
Baseball
Curling

Bowling
Ice hockey
Lacrosse
Swimming: 100 meters
   and less
Field hockey
Football
Golf
Gymnastics
Racquetball

you can benefit from cross-training with sports that are 50% or more fueled by anaerobic glycolysis, such as

Swimming: 200+ meters
Cycling: match sprints
Tennis
Track: 800–1,600 meters
Basketball*

Dance*
Wrestling
Mountain climbing*
Synchronized swimming
Laser sailing

or you can train the endurance system with sports that are 50% or more fueled by the aerobic system, such as

Cycling: 4,000-meter
   pursuit, criteria,
   25–100K
Running: 3 miles or more
Skiing: cross-country

Swimming: 1,500–1,650
   meters and long distance
Triathlon: swim, bike, run
Rowing
Kayaking

Endurance athletes can also benefit by training the power and speed systems for strength and faster times for running, swimming, cycling, skiing, and rowing.

*These sports are a blend of the aerobic and anaerobic systems, depending on duration and intensity.

Not surprisingly, the energy needs of vegetarian athletes also vary according to the athlete's body size, weight, and composition, as well as gender, sport, and training program. (In chapter 2 you will learn how these factors and exercise increase the amount of calories you use daily.) In a recent study, caloric intake of vegetarian athletes was shown to be about 11% higher than in meat-eating athletes. Some explanations may be increased appetites of low-fat, high-carbohydrate vegetarian eaters; the increased metabolic efficiency of vegetarian athletes; or perhaps that vegetarians can just eat more than other athletes. As an added benefit, while we're eating more nutritious food, we're getting more vitamins, minerals, and other substances the body needs for peak sports performance.

According to the one-day dietary analysis of the spotlight athletes profiled in this book, they consumed between 1,100 and 5,028 calories per day and have no difficulty in meeting energy and other nutrient needs except when traveling (more on this in chapter 10).

Carbohydrates

The plant-based, high-carbohydrate diet has special advantages for endurance athletes. For years, solid research has shown the benefits of high-carbohydrate diets for sports performance as well as the detriments of low-carbohydrate diets. High-carbohydrate diets maximize muscle and liver glycogen stores, optimize performance during prolonged moderate exercise intensity, and improve intermittent, short-duration, and high-intensity exercise (see chapter 3).

Carbohydrates benefit sport performance because

1. Liver and muscle glycogen are the predominant fuels for continuous running, swimming, and cycling and extended, mixed anaerobic/aerobic sports such as soccer, basketball, and repeated interval running.

2. Exhaustion during prolonged hard exercise is related to low muscle glycogen stores.

3. Low carbohydrate stores prevent maintenance of high-energy output. Because fat cannot fuel high-intensity exercise, a high-carbohydrate diet is essential for System 1a– and 1b–level (power system and anaerobic glycolysis) sprint sports.

4. Muscle glycogen stores fluctuate and deplete rapidly during

strenuous training. No matter what your diet, a two-hour workout can easily use up valuable fuels. However, a high-carbohydrate, plant-based diet can help to postpone depletion. Training at 60 to 80% of your VO2 maximum aerobic capacity (see box below) will lead to depletion after 100 to 120 minutes. Exercise at 80 to 95% VO2max will lead to depletion even sooner. A consistent plant-based, high-carbohydrate diet of 70% of total calories or 8 to 10 grams of carbohydrates per kilogram of body weight is guaranteed to make a difference for daily endurance-trained athletes.

5. The body adapts to maximizing muscle and liver glycogen through endurance training. Well-trained athletes can even manipulate rest and diet by using a regimen called "glycogen loading" the week before a long-distance event to cause the muscles to overcompensate with extra-high levels of glycogen—nearly doubling the levels of those untrained. (See pages 53–55 for more information on glycogen loading.)

Understanding VO2max

Regular exercise trains your system to transport more oxygen-rich blood to your organs and muscles. One convenient measure of aerobic fitness is called the VO2max. It is the maximum amount of oxygen that the body is able to use for the purpose of producing energy. There are two ways to calculate your own VO2max. The more precise way is taking a treadmill test while connected to a tube that measures exhaled gases as you gradually push yourself to a maximum output. You can also use estimates to find your target pace. Although heart rate and VO2max are not the same, multiplying your maximum heart rate (estimated by subtracting your age from 220) by a certain percentage (say .90) corresponds in this case to 90% of maximum. Research has shown that VO2max is one way to predict performance in aerobically based events such as distance running, road cycling, Nordic skiing, and triathlon.

Endurance training also helps athletes use more fats as fuel, thereby sparing glycogen, at any exercise intensity. In fact, with endurance training, fats (triglycerides) stored within the muscles increase by as much as 83%. That makes fats more available as an energy source. Vegetarian athletes therefore have an even greater advantage when consuming their high-carbohydrate diets and endurance training or cross-"aerobic" training for any sport.

Protein

Protein needs vary according to many factors, including age, calorie intake, gender, and level of training (see chapter 4). Inadequate intakes of carbohydrate and calories increase protein requirements. During prolonged endurance exercise, such as the marathon, ultra-marathon, and ironman distance triathlon, athletes with low glycogen stores metabolize twice as much protein to meet carbohydrate needs.

On the average, vegetarian diets contain about 12.5% of total calories from protein, and vegan diets contain 11%. Collectively, the athletes profiled in this book get about 20% of their calories from protein (17% for the vegans). These values exceed the World Health Organization (WHO) dietary protein recommendations for nonactive individuals. As you can see, vegetarian eating programs can easily meet protein requirements through grains, beans, nuts, soy, and vegetables.

Athletes who are semi-, lacto-, or lacto-ovo-vegetarian usually consume enough protein because of the inclusion of milk, cheese, eggs, fish, and poultry products. The greatest challenge for consuming enough protein comes when food options are limited (which is common when traveling) and training programs that require additional amounts of protein.

Endurance- and strength-trained athletes, bodybuilders, growing athletes, and those with high training levels and low calorie intakes need to include more protein than other athletes do. High-protein formulas and foods are discussed in chapter 4.

Fat

Research suggests that athletes do not benefit from more than 30% fat from total calorie intake. That's good, because vegetarians generally do not have to worry about consuming too much fat. Most plant-based foods are naturally low in fat. If anything, some athletes have been known to obsess over the desire to consume too little fat. While low-fat diets have been used in clinical settings to manage heart disease, obesity, and other chronic conditions, they have not been useful in sports diets. In fact, very low-fat diets may hinder performance (see chapter 5).

The athletes in this book consume approximately 6 to 28% of their total calories from fat, despite recent trendy sports diet recommendations that *suggest* greater amounts of fat, such as 40/30/30 (see chapter 10) and the Zone. Although plant-based foods are naturally low-fat, some vegetarians consume too much fat, saturated fat, and cholesterol by choosing high-fat dairy products and fish or preparing foods with high-fat sauces and ingredients such as oil and dressings. In this book, Chef Hanners has created low-fat, healthier versions of favorite traditionally high-fat vegetarian recipes such as Hummus (page 24), and Roasted Eggplant Pomodoro (page 25).

Vitamin and Mineral Needs

Vegetarian diets can easily provide the requirements for most vitamins; however, riboflavin (B_2) and B_{12} are potential exceptions. The athletes here had exceptional intakes of most of the vitamins and minerals, with the exception of vitamin D and biotin. Low levels of vitamin D may be the result of eliminating fortified dairy and fish from their diets. Biotin intakes may be reduced due to the elimination of egg yolk and liver from their diets. The vitamin and mineral intakes for all 17 athletes (including me) appear in chapter 7.

Studies have suggested that riboflavin needs may increase in marginally deficient individuals who begin a new exercise program. Diets of strict vegetarians tend to be lower in riboflavin, unless enough dairy or plant sources are consumed daily. Active vegetarians who avoid dairy products can include the fortified plant-based sources of riboflavin provided on pages 202–203, in the recipe guide on page 135, and those discussed in chapter 7.

Vitamin B_{12} is critical to the maintenance of cells in the blood and nervous systems. Because humans primarily get vitamin B_{12} through dietary animal sources, vegans need to include vitamin B_{12}-fortified products such as those listed on page 135, have a fortified sports bar or shake, or take a supplement to prevent a deficiency. Semi- and lacto-ovo-vegetarians generally do not need vitamin B_{12} supplements because milk and other dairy products as well as fish contain adequate amounts.

Antioxidants. Evidence suggests that vitamins C, E, and beta-carotene may protect against exercise-induced oxidative stress (see chapter 7). Several studies have summarized the potential benefits of antioxidant supplements to protect against free radical production. Vegetarian athletes may have an advantage since antioxidants are readily obtained from a diet rich in vegetables, nuts, seeds, and vegetable oils. The vegetarian athletes in this book get an abundance of antioxidants naturally, but several, including Dave Scott, Chris Campbell, Craig Heath, Gary Gromet, and myself, take antioxidant supplements regularly.

Calcium. According to the Recommended Dietary Allowances (RDAs), calcium recommendations for active men and women are the same as for normal individuals. Dietary calcium intake influences the body's balance by only 11%. Urinary calcium excretion accounts for 51% of losses and is affected by dietary protein, sodium, and possibly phosphoric acid intakes. As a result, some dairy- or egg-limiting vegetarians and vegans may have lower calcium requirements due to lower dietary intakes of protein (especially animal protein) and sodium, which increase renal excretion.

Athletes with low calcium intakes, especially amenorrheic (non-menstruating) women, are at risk for stress fractures and low bone density. An estimated 20 to 50% of competitive female athletes have amenorrhea. Although the cause of athletic amenorrhea has not been determined, several investigators have shown that female distance runners have an insufficient calorie intake for their training levels. This energy drain, or an eating disorder masked by vegetarianism, may be a contributing factor in athletic amenorrhea.

In one study of eight meat-free amenorrheic athletes, the average calorie intake was 1,582 calories per day. Iron, magnesium, folic acid, riboflavin, and zinc intakes were one-third of the RDAs. Although a number of reports suggest that vegetarian athletes tend to have more menstrual problems, others have reported that adequately nourished female vegetarian athletes menstruate normally when compared with the general population.

Researchers have reasoned that hormonal precursors and essential minerals such as zinc and iron could be affected by reduced intake of meat, especially in runners. Female vegetarians have also been found to have lower levels of circulating estrogen. This may be due to their high-fiber, low-fat diets. Since a calcium intake of 1,500 milligrams per day is needed to retain calcium balance in women with low circulating estrogens, higher calcium intakes may be required for amenorrheic as well as postmenopausal athletes.

Iron. All athletes are at risk for iron depletion and iron deficiency anemia. Not only is this unhealthy, but low iron levels, even without anemia, have been shown to decrease performance. Iron loss is common in some heavily training athletes due to

▶ gastrointestinal bleeding

▶ heavy sweating

▶ blood cell breakdown

▶ insufficient iron intake or reduced absorption

Studies have shown that female vegetarian runners consume similar amounts of iron as nonvegetarian athletes, but retain less. This may be due in part to the fact that most vegetarian foods are sources of non-heme iron, which has a lower absorption rate (2 to 20%) than heme iron from meat products (15 to 35%) (see chapter 7 to learn about heme and non-heme iron). Three of the athletes profiled in this book take an iron supplement, though their diets do not warrant its use. Tips for "ironing up" vegetarian meals with non-heme-rich recipes are in chapters 7 and 8.

Zinc. Although the zinc status of vegetarians has not been well researched, several studies have reported decreased zinc levels in heavily training athletes. Pay attention to your zinc intake because plant-based diets contain high concentrations of phytates, which can inhibit zinc absorption (see chapter 7).

Creatine

Creatine monohydrate is a hot supplement among athletes, particularly vegetarian athletes. Several of the athletes in this book take a creatine supplement. Most of the creatine in the body is found in muscle. It serves as an energy backup to ATP in System 1a anaerobic sports. Vegetarians get little creatine because it is found primarily in muscle tissue. Meat eaters get about 2 grams per day.

Although creatine can be synthesized from blood, amino acid precursors, and skeletal muscle, levels have been shown to be lower in vegetarians than nonvegetarians. Therefore, vegetarians may benefit from creatine supplements even more than nonvegetarians (see chapter 8).

As this overview of sports nutrition has shown, there are few unique needs imposed by a plant-based diet. In fact, a nutrient-dense vegetarian diet is ideal for sports and daily fitness activities. Knowing your energy needs in order to understand how to incorporate plant-based foods into your daily training program is a necessity. You can be certain to meet your daily dietary needs by using the Foundation Food Lists, recipes, and food tips throughout this book to get the "biggest bang" from every meal and snack.

Now, grab one of the athletes' favorite snacks listed below and a liter of water to fuel you through chapter 2, "Nutrition Prescription for Sport."

▶ VEGETARIAN SPORTS NUTRITION GUIDE ◀
Athletes' Favorite Snacks

HIGH-CARBOHYDRATE (MORE THAN 50% CALORIES FROM CARBOHYDRATES)
Athletes

Carrot sticks*	Popcorn
German bread	Chips/salsa
Walnut bagels	Kabochia squash*
Rice cakes	Radishes*
Saltine crackers	Corn tortillas
Pretzels	

continued

▶ *Athletes' Favorite Snacks (continued)*

Author

Dried pea snack*

Figs rolled in coconut*

Dole or Frozfruit bars

Fruit salad with dried
strawberries and
blueberries*

Organic fat-free yogurt

Oat bran pretzels

Dried bananas

Fresh fruit

Fresh fruit smoothie

Fat-free soy cheese with apple

Raisin-cinnamon mochi

Mountain Lift Bars

Whole wheat organic
tortillas, lightly toasted

Balance Shake

HIGH-CARBOHYDRATE, HIGH-SIMPLE SUGAR
(MORE THAN 8 GRAMS OF SUGAR PER SERVING [2 TSP.])

Athletes

Cherry licorice

PowerBars

Sweet potatoes

Apples

Fruit

Banana

Fruit shakes

Health nut cookies

Figs

Oranges

Raisins

Cinnamon grahams

Dole fruit bars

Cinnamon applesauce

Author

Fresh fruit smoothies

Frozen yogurt

Hain's vanilla and
chocolate rice cakes

Natural fruit rollups

Dried fruit

Japanese rice cakes
(Sanshoku Dango)

Häagen-Dazs sorbets

Licorice

HIGH-FAT (MORE THAN 5 GRAMS PER SERVING)

Athletes

Peanuts

Candy bars

Corn chips

Peanut butter and jelly

Ice cream

Chocolate

Trail mix

Oil-popped popcorn

continued

▶ *Athletes' Favorite Snacks (continued)*

Author

Soy nuts with raisins   Trail mix with soy nuts, dried pea
Green tea ice cream   snack, and dried cranberries

HIGH-PROTEIN (MORE THAN 10 GRAMS OF PROTEIN PER SERVING)

Edamame (boiled soybeans   Dried pea snack
    in husk)   PowerBars
Roasted soybeans   Power Chips
Balance bars   Fat-free soy cheese
Frozen protein shakes   Met-Rx Bars
Parillo Bars   Ginger/shoya tea with kuzu

*Contains fiber, spices, or too much fat to consume 1–4 hours before running or
triathlon competitions.

Hanners' Hummus

Makes 14 servings

---

4 cups fresh garbanzo beans
2 lemons, zest and juice
6 cloves garlic, minced
½ bunch parsley, chopped fine
salt and pepper to taste

In a food processor, blend the garbanzo beans until a smooth
paste begins to form. Add the other ingredients and continue
to blend until they are well-distributed in the mixture. It can
be served with baked pita chips, bagel chips, or rice crackers.

▶ Nutrients per serving: 217 calories, 11 grams protein, 36 grams
   carbohydrates, 3 grams fat, 0.5 grams monounsaturated fat, 0.2
   grams sugar, 0.2 grams fiber
▶ Dietary composition: 21% protein, 65% carbohydrates, 14% fat
▶ *Vegetarian Sports Nutrition Guide* food servings: 2.5 grains, 1 fat
▶ Good source of potassium, phosphorus, and iron

Hanners' Roasted Eggplant Pomodoro

Makes 1 serving

Great for pasta as alternative to red sauce!

1 full ripe eggplant
1 tsp olive oil
5 plum tomatoes, chopped roughly
1/2 bunch basil, chopped
1 tsp balsamic vinegar
1/2 lemon, juiced
pinch salt and pepper

Split eggplant in half lengthwise. Make deep diamond-shaped scores into eggplant. Lay face up on cooking sheet. Drizzle olive oil onto eggplant and season. Bake at 350 degrees F approximately 40 minutes. When cool, remove skin.

In food processor, add remaining ingredients. Blend until a smooth sauce is formed. Serve over any pasta, including a fettuccine or quinoa penne.

▶ Nutrients per serving: 213 calories, 6.5 grams protein, 39 grams carbohydrates, 7 grams fat, 4 grams monounsaturated fat, 1 gram linoleic fat, 18 grams sugar, 11 grams fiber.

▶ Dietary composition: 11% protein, 64% carbohydrates, 25% fat

▶ *Vegetarian Sports Nutrition Guide* food servings: 3 cups vegetables, 1 fat

▶ Good source of vitamins A, C, and K, folate, and potassium; moderate source of vitamins B_1, B_2, B_3, B_6, E, and pantothenic acid, biotin, magnesium, iron, and copper.

Spotlight Athlete

Ruth Heidrich, Ph.D.
Six-Time Ironwoman, Marathoner, and
USA Track and Field Master's Champion

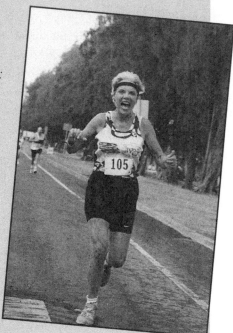

Age: 64

17 years vegan

Reason for becoming vegetarian:
"After being diagnosed with breast cancer in 1982, I joined a research study to determine the effect of a ten percent fat vegan diet on reversing breast cancer. I have stayed with the program since that time."

Advantages of being vegetarian: "Faster, better endurance and recovery time and rapid bowel-transit time!"

Challenges to being vegetarian: "None!"

Alcohol: none

Supplements: none

Favorite pre-event meal: brown rice, kale, banana, and black-strap molasses mixed and microwaved for 2 minutes (see page 37)

Favorite snacks: air-popped popcorn, sweet potatoes, apples, and carrot sticks

Favorite one-pot meal: Ruth's Ironwoman Pho (Vietnamese soup, page 149)

2

Nutrition Prescription for Sport: Calculating Energy Needs

A S A TWO-TIME OLYMPIC WRESTLER, 1992 Olympic bronze medalist, world champion, and four-time World Cup champion, Chris Campbell can attest to the fact that a vegetarian diet can meet all your energy and nutrient needs and then some.

Not only was he the oldest Olympic medalist in a combat sport in the 1992 Olympic Games, he accomplished this after a five-year break from competing. He was the first wrestler to take an extended leave and return to the sport to win a medal, at age 38 no less. Chris is now executive director of USA Boxing and married with three children. He credits his accomplishments to a diet that prevents clogged arteries and other damage that slows the body down. He feels "almost as supple and fast" as he was at age 30, before his first retirement.

The advantages he finds to being a vegetarian include a reduction in dietary fat and the ability to maintain a healthy weight for nineteen years. Being a vegetarian allowed him to use energy for training instead of for processing meat. Even though his friends would "balloon up" in weight and get "real puffy" after not training for a while, he avoided that syndrome by remaining a lacto-ovo-vegetarian.

Chris became a vegetarian after doing his own research on maximizing athletic performance for the 1980 Olympic Games. His quest led him to the conclusion that the vegetarian diet would allow his body to be at its peak. "I would not have the physical zapping of strength associated with having the body handle meat," Chris said.

After being a vegetarian for four years, his reasons for staying a vegetarian changed dramatically. It became a moral and spiritual issue. He no longer believed he had the right to take another animal's life to continue his own. The only challenges he has faced as a vegetarian are on the road. For instance, "When I would travel to Russia, trying to get a vegetarian meal was tough. I would eat a lot of bread," he said.

His ethnic roots do not influence his daily intake of a variety of beans, rice, oatmeal, apples, and other foods. His foods tend to have a mix of Indian, Moroccan, Chinese, and Japanese flavors. His favorite pre-event meal is beans and rice or pancakes, and favorite snacks include apples and chocolate. He drinks wine or beer just twice weekly and supplements with a multivitamin, vitamin E, B complex, and Alacers E-Mergen-C (see chapter 8). Chris offers his favorite one-pot energizing oatmeal dish at the end of this chapter.

Energy Prescription for Athletes

It is common practice for wrestlers like Chris to restrict food and fluids to compete in weight classes below their normal weight. Wrestlers call this technique "making weight," which they say provides a competitive edge in performance. Athletes such as Ben Mathews, Debbie Stephens, and others (see chapters 3 and 10) have turned to vegetarianism as a way to meet the best competitive weights for their sports. Although vegetarians, through their low-fat, less calorically dense diets, may have an easier time meeting their ideal body weights, there are many other factors that make this seemingly simple system very complex.

Regardless of your sport, weight maintenance results from achieving an energy balance that matches total energy intake from food to total energy expenditure. Daily energy expenditure is comprised of

▶ resting metabolic rate or Basal Energy Expenditure (BEE)

▶ activity, or energy expenditure

▶ Specific Dynamic Action (SDA) or Thermic Effect of Feeding

▶ adaptive thermogenesis

Resting Metabolic Rate or Basal Energy Expenditure

The basal metabolic rate (BMR) accounts for 60 to 75% of the body's total energy requirement. It is activity required for the basic maintenance of body life and function, awake, in a steady state, unfed, in a neutral warm environment, at complete rest.

Sound simple? It's not.

There are many individual factors that influence this number. First of all, it is closely related to the amount of lean muscle (total weight − % of body fat in weight) the athlete has. Factors that influence lean muscle weight are age, sex, body composition, and genetics. Someone like Chris and other elite athletes with a low body-fat percentage can use up more than 19% additional calories than the average person for Basal Energy Expenditure (BEE). Heredity can account for up to 40% of individual variation. Other factors that may influence BEE are listed below.

▶ Factors that May Affect Basal Metabolic Rate ◀	
Age	The younger one is, the more calories one uses at rest.
Height	Tall, thin people have higher resting metabolic rates.
Growth	Children and pregnant women have higher basal rates.
Body composition	More muscle means more calories used at rest.
Fever	Fever raises BMR.
Stress	Stress hormones raise BMR.
Environment	Very hot or cool climates can raise BMR (at least initially).
Temperature	Cold and heat raise BMR.
Fasting/starvation	Fasting lowers BMR.
Malnutrition	Malnutrition lowers BMR.
Thyroxine	The thyroid hormone thyroxine controls the internal calorie regulator; the less thyroxine produced, the more sluggish metabolism is.
Thermic effect of food	In leaner people, metabolism speeds up after consuming food, while in obese people, no change occurs.

Activity and Energy Expenditure

All daily activities and exercise can contribute to changing the BEE calorie needs by about 15 to 30%. Training changes and adaptation to long-term training can influence resting metabolic rate as well as the rate at which your body processes food, called the Specific Dynamic Action of Food (SDA) or Thermic Effect of Feeding (TEF).

Exercise causes both acute and long-term effects on energy expenditure. The greater the energy output, the greater the overall daily energy expenditure. Excess Postexercise Oxygen Consumption (EPOC), the amount of calories one uses after exercise, has long been established. Studies have shown that the duration of EPOC may last one to twenty-four hours postexercise, increasing the metabolic rate from 1 to 25%. Recent information shows that most of the EPOC effect is within the first hour and greater with higher-intensity, longer-duration exercise. An Olympic distance triathlon, 10K road race, or cross-country ski race would meet the intensity (over 70% of maximum heart rate) and duration (over 60 minutes) criteria.

While the total EPOC expenditure is normally only 0.7 to 71.7 calories, over time it can account for up to 500 calories each week and help maintain energy balance. This may be due to the body using more fat as exercise continues and muscle glycogen stores become depleted. Fatty acid levels may remain elevated for up to 24 hours postexercise. This sparing of glucose (carbohydrates) for energy may help to replenish muscle glycogen stores.

Although the physiological mechanisms have not been determined, resynthesis of ATP, creatine phosphate, protein, and glycogen may also contribute to the energy equation. Metabolic hormones, calcium concentrations, sodium activity, and body temperature will also influence EPOC.

The level of training may also significantly influence resting metabolic rate. Consistent exercise has also been shown to increase metabolic rate. It is also possible that BEE is only higher when endurance training is complemented by a high-calorie diet.

This may also be coupled with a high caloric turnover (increased energy intake and expenditure), which effects enzymatic activity, or an accumulative EPOC effect of exercise intensity, duration, frequency, and the thermic effect of meals taken postexercise.

Therefore, since increasing physical activity may help to expend more calories, it's logical that spending more time exercising would make losing or maintaining a specific weight easier. Exercise does this by diminishing the appetite as a result of elevated body temperatures, increasing the BEE and the thermic effect of food. Oddly, the overall effectiveness may be gender-dependent. In one study, hormones that stimulate fat breakdown were 66% greater in males while just 46% greater in females after completing a twenty-week aerobic exercise program.

The Influence of Exercise on Food

In lean individuals, one session of mild to moderate exercise has been shown to exert a potentiating effect on the Specific Dynamic Action of Food (SDA). However, leaner individuals are more sensitive than the obese to thermogenic hormones.

The timing of exercise relative to the meal may also influence the magnitude of the thermic effect. Studies have shown that leaner individuals use more calories for SDA when meals are consumed before exercise, while in the obese it's greatest after. So if you want to lose weight, hold off on snacking until after the exercise session.

Research has had mixed results regarding the influence of chronic exercise on SDA, still a controversial issue. In a cross-sectional study of males covering a wide range of intensity capabilities and endurance training levels, SDA was shown to be greatest in the moderately trained, when compared with highly trained and untrained individuals. Reasons for this include the influence of hormones and genetics. An elevated BEE in the highly trained may also disguise the portion of SDA elevation.

Specific Dynamic Action of Food (SDA)

The SDA accounts for about 10% of energy needs. It is used for the digestion, absorption, transport, metabolism, and storage of food. The caloric content and composition of a meal, nutritional state, individual genotype, fitness level, and the antecedent diet of the athlete all influence the SDA.

Adaptive Thermogenesis

Adaptive thermogenesis is a change in heat production within the body without a change in activity levels. It ultimately affects daily energy expenditure as a result of environmental and/or physiological stresses such as exposure to cold or under- or overeating. Changes in both BEE and SDA, as a result of training, play a role in adaptive thermogenesis.

Dietary Factors

Both quantity and dietary composition may influence energy expenditure. Undernutrition causes a decrease in expenditure. This serves as a protective mechanism to prevent excessive energy losses during periods of fasting. The degree of restriction and length of training on restricted diets influences the capability of exercise to reverse the decrease in BEE. While severe calorie restriction of 800 calories or less may inhibit successful weight loss, endurance exercise on a restricted diet may prevent a decline in resting metabolic rate. Animal studies suggest a 10-week time lapse before decreases in metabolic rates were statistically significant. Overnutrition causes an increase in energy expenditure due to changes in the SDA and hormones.

Dietary composition may also influence these changes, since humans have only a limited ability to convert excess dietary carbohydrate to fat. For instance, even a 500-gram-carbohydrate meal (2,000 calories) results in maximum glycogen storage, an elevated rate of carbohydrate usage, and a decrease in the rate of fat metabolism.

Metabolic Cost

Protein and carbohydrates are vital to daily metabolic functions. Since the body has limited capacity to store these nutrients, the rate at which the body uses them varies with dietary intake.

The calorie "cost" of storing carbohydrate is greater than that of storing fat. That means that the body's limited capacity to store carbohydrate in liver and muscle, to about 1,600 to 2,400 calories (400–600 grams), is cheaper than converting it to fat. The maintenance of fat balance within the body is not subject to the same mechanisms.

High-fat diets (59% total calories) have been associated with reduced energy expenditure. Since fat is used or stored in response to changes in calorie intake, excessive amounts will cause an accumulation of excess body fat. That means that for the same amount of calories, fattier foods cause more stored body fat than carbohydrate (plant-based) foods.

Chronic high-fat diets have also been shown to change protein and carbohydrate metabolism. Healthy, lean individuals on high-fat diets (84%) for four weeks at maintenance calorie levels use less glucose (sugar) for fuel. This demonstrates the body's ability to spare carbohydrate at all costs to adapt the body's metabolism to the predominant nutrient consumed in the diet.

So Many Formulas, So Little Time

There are many ways to calculate energy (calorie) needs for the active individual. From simple to complex "guesstimates" of indirect measurement, this is how sports nutritionists calculate dietary needs outside of the lab. Most rely on the same factors for calculating the body's daily calorie needs: Basal Energy Metabolism (BEE), activity, and Specific Dynamic Action of Food (SDA).

Since exercise influences a cumulative effect on BEE, SDA, and active thermogenesis, it is challenging to calculate an accurate energy equation for athletes without precise measurements.

In the early part of the twentieth century, numerous studies of basal energy expenditure were conducted under the direction of Francis G. Benedict. Prediction equation studies from these formulas were developed from these studies. The Harris–Benedict equations remain the most common method for calculating BEE for clinical and research purposes since they have a sound physiological basis for use and can be applied over a wide range of ages and body types.

Calculate your desirable weight and body fat from the formula in chapter 10. Then use those numbers in these BEE calculations.

The Harris–Benedict equations are

Men: BEE (calories/day) =
         $65 + (13.40 \times \text{weight}) + (4.96 \times \text{height}) - (5.82 \times \text{age})$

Women: BEE (calories/day) =
         $447 + (9.25 \times \text{weight}) + (3.10 \times \text{height}) - (4.33 \times \text{age})$

To calculate the needs of inactive to moderately active individuals, this formula is fine. However, research has shown a better method for endurance-trained athletes. This formula, called the Cunningham equation, is more accurate because it is based on fat-free mass versus body mass. The following information will help you to calculate your energy needs according to this equation.

▶ Calculating Daily Energy (Calorie) Needs ◀

Step One
Using the Cunningham equation for endurance training, you need to find out your percentage of body fat composition from a certified fitness professional to ensure accuracy (see Appendix C).

BEE = 500 calories + 22 × (Fat Free Mass in kilograms body weight)*

*Fat Free Mass (kg) is Total weight – % body fat weight.

Step Two
Add the amount of calories used for training (energy expenditure).

There are many charts you can use from a variety of exercise physiology textbooks to give you the amount of calories you use for a variety of activities, at various body weights and speeds. Some of these figures are provided for you below.

Energy Expenditure Estimates

ACTIVITY		CALORIES/HOUR, KG/BW		
		50 kg (110 lbs.)	70 kg (154 lbs.)	90 kg (198 lbs.)
Cycling		150–400	210–560	270–720
Running				
7 MPH	1.68/kg/mile			
8 MPH	1.66/kg/mile			
9 MPH	1.64/kg/mile			
10 MPH	1.63/kg/mile			
Sitting		66	92	120
Swimming: crawl				
Females	260–360 cal/mile			
Males	360–500 cal/mile			
Walking		240	307	437
Weightlifting		258	361	470

continued

▶ *Calculating Daily Energy (Calorie) Needs (continued)*

Step Three

Add together the sums of step one and step two and multiply by 10% to account for the energy spent for the complete digestion and metabolism of food. Add all three steps together to get a "guesstimate" of indirect calorimetry, in other words, an estimate of your daily calorie needs.

Total calories needed per day = BEE + Activity + SDA

The total amount of calories you have added together is the amount you need to maintain the weight that you have designated as your present or ideal body weight.

You can now use your personal calorie prescription throughout the book as you apply it to calculating your carbohydrate, protein, and fat requirements. After you finish calculating your energy needs, enjoy a bowl of Chris's Wrestling Oats or Ruth's Pre-Race (PR) Porridge, prepared in a similar fashion. You can also prepare one of the other athletes' favorite one-pot dishes highlighted on their Spotlight Athlete profiles and on the charts in chapter 9. Recipes appear throughout the book.

Spotlight Athlete

Chris Campbell

Olympic wrestler, 1992 Olympic bronze medalist, world champion, and four-time World Cup champion

Age: 44

Married, three children

19 years lacto-ovo-vegetarian

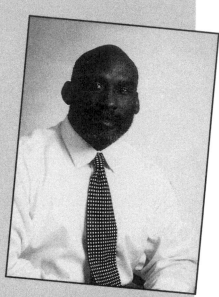

Reason for becoming vegetarian: "Before the 1980 Olympic games I was researching all the issues relating to maximum athletic performance. The research led me to the conclusion that the vegetarian diet would allow my body to be at its peak. I would not have the physical zapping of strength associated with having the body handle meat. . . . After I was a vegetarian for four years, my reasons for staying a vegetarian were different. I no longer believed I had the right to take another animal's life to continue my life. It became a moral and spiritual issue."

Advantages of being vegetarian: "Handling meat consumes the body's energy. Being a vegetarian allows me to use that energy for training. In addition, my fat intake is reduced. Therefore, it is easier for me to maintain my weight. Many of my friends would balloon up in weight and get real puffy after not training for a while. That would never happen to me. I have maintained my ideal weight for the entire nineteen years . . . In addition, I was the oldest Olympic medalist in a combat sport in the 1992 Olympic Games. This was after I had taken five years off from competing. No one had ever taken that much time off and won a medal, especially at age thirty-seven, one month shy of turning thirty-eight. I believe this was possible because I did not have the accumulated artery and other damages that slow the body down. I was almost as supple and fast as I was before I retired when I was thirty."

Challenges to being a vegetarian: "When I would travel to Russia, trying to get a vegetarian meal was tough. I would eat a lot of bread."

Alcohol: wine or beer twice weekly

Supplements: E-Mergen-C, Vitamin E and B complex, and a multivitamin

Favorite pre-event meal: beans and rice or pancakes

Favorite snacks: apples and chocolate

Favorite one-pot meal: Campbell's Wrestling Oatmeal (similar to Ruth's Porridge; see below)

Ruth's Pre-Race (PR) Porridge

Makes 1 serving

(Similar to Chris Campbell's pre-event favorite "Wrestling Oats")

—

1 cup cooked long-grain rice
1 cup kale
1 banana
1 tbsp molasses

—

Take the cup of cooked long-grain rice. Mix in the kale. Add the sliced banana. Fold in the molasses to cover all ingredients in mixture.

▶ Nutrients per serving: 408 calories, 8.5 grams protein, 90 grams carbohydrates, 3 grams fat, 29 grams sugar, 9 grams fiber

▶ Dietary composition: 8% protein, 86% carbohydrates, 6% fat

3

Carbohydrates: The Sports Nutrition Base

BUILDING A SOLID NUTRITIONAL BASE with carbohydrates is second nature for the spotlight athletes featured in this chapter. Jane Welzel, 2:33 marathoner and 1990 National Marathon Champion, and Ben Mathews, masters marathon sensation, both appreciate the critical role of sustaining energy levels for training and racing the marathon distance. There is no doubt in their minds that carbohydrates play a pivotal role before, during, and after their performance on race day.

At 43, there is no room for nutritional deficiencies in the life of a marathoner. Jane Welzel has ensured her eating success by becoming a lacto-ovo-vegetarian 23 years ago while raising animals and not being able to "make that leap from pet to dinner." She sees the advantage of being a vegetarian as guaranteeing a healthy diet of easy-to-digest foods between workouts.

Jane starts the day with a mocha espresso before her morning workout. The value of the caffeine, chocolate, and skim milk before her 60- to 75-minute run is highlighted in this chapter and chapter 8. The rest of her day includes four more snack/meals, which are composed of seitan, tofu cheese, tofu, bread, crackers, rice, and vegetables. After two more workouts in midday and late afternoon, she enjoys a glass of wine with dinner and some jelly beans for dessert.

Still in top form after completing eighty marathons, Ben Mathews is any young or master athlete's dream. As a full-time certified public accountant (CPA), he finds time to squeeze in two training sessions daily, one ten-mile-plus running workout and one evening swim, while adhering to a macrobiotic diet for the last seven years. Unlike other vegetarian programs, macrobiotics requires lifestyle, food preparation, and other changes that consume additional time on his "marathon" days. Being married to a macrobiotic wife and race walker helps alleviate some of the effort necessary to prepare special macrobiotic meals. His four children, now grown, live in other parts of the country.

While Jane and Ben take no medications, Jane differs from Ben when it comes to a daily glass of wine. Jane also takes supplements to complement her meal program, while Ben relies on his food to do the work.

Jane's and Ben's favorite foods, prerace meals, and snacks are discussed throughout this chapter on carbohydrates, the sports nutrition base.

A Simple and Complex Issue

Both anaerobic and aerobic sports rely on the availability of carbohydrate fuel. Both simple and complex carbohydrates contribute to the primary fuel needed for sport. Jane and Ben represent two outstanding marathon runners who rely on carbohydrates for their primary energy source.

Simple carbohydrates are called mono- and disaccharides, in the form of glucose, fructose, galactose, sucrose, maltose, and lactose. Simple sugars are associated with sweet foods, honey, candy, desserts, and fruits. Sport bars and drinks also contain simple carbohydrates for quick energy. Complex carbohydrates are glycogen (animal and human stored form), starch (plant form), and fibers. The foods in this category include pastas, cereals, breads, crackers, rice, potatoes, vegetables, and fruits.

Green plants make carbohydrates through photosynthesis in the presence of chlorophyll and sunlight. In the process, water is absorbed by the plant's roots, donating its hydrogen and oxygen. The carbon dioxide gas absorbed in the plant's leaves donates carbon and oxygen. Water and carbon dioxide combine to yield the simplest sugar, glucose.

Starch is the plant's storage form for glucose. As the plant matures, starch is stored in its seeds for the growth of plants next season. The human body also stores starch, called glycogen, in the liver and muscles. Another complex sugar called fiber contributes the supporting structures of its leaves, stems, and seeds. Some fibers are water-soluble and some are not. These differences have varying physical effects on the body. These fibers cannot be digested by humans and pass through the system, assisting in facilitating the movement of food through the gastrointestinal tract. Ruth has pointed out that one of the advantages of being a vegetarian is the "rapid bowel-transit time."

Top Gun

Glucose is the preferred fuel for most body functions. It is the major fuel for nerve cells, the brain, and exercise. The World Health Organization recommends a complex carbohydrate intake of 50 to 75% of total calorie consumption, and simple carbohydrate consumption of approximately 10% or less of total consumption.

This means that an athlete consuming 2,000 calories per day would benefit from a range of 1,000 to 1,500 calories (250–375 grams) of complex carbohydrates, with only 100 to 150 calories (25–37 grams) of simple sugars. Calculations for this formula are located at the end of the chapter.

WHO and other health care organizations recommend limiting simple sugars because these foods are often lower in protein, vitamins, minerals, and fiber (e.g., candy, fruit "drinks," and soda); higher in fats and saturated fats (e.g., cake, candy, and ice cream); and displace the consumption of nutrient-rich foods from the diet.

That doesn't mean that Jane and other athletes who consume substantial complex carbohydrates and train regularly can't "have their cake and eat it, too!" The sugars are still an energy source and provide a mental boost or relief from the seriousness and intensity of training.

On the other hand, complex carbohydrates are more beneficial because they

▶ promote a feeling of fullness with meals, helping reduce the total amount of food consumed

▶ prevent dehydration by absorbing water when they're consumed (about 3 grams water for every gram of carbohydrate consumed)

▶ reduce calorie intake by displacing calorie-rich, high-fat sweets

I personally feel and perform better when I consume a high-complex-carbohydrate diet. Several athletes in this book, including myself, enjoy beans, tortillas, mochi, potatoes, peas, and hot multigrain cereals for our daily favorite high-carb choices.

The additional benefits of getting a variety of whole grains, vegetables, and fruits are the blend of water-soluble and insoluble fibers. These fibers may help athletes and others by

▶ preventing constipation and hemorrhoids

▶ preventing bacterial infection of the appendix (i.e., appendicitis)

▶ stimulating the muscles of the gastrointestinal tract, retaining their health and tone, and possibly preventing diverticulitis, a disease of the GI tract

▶ improving the body's handling of sugar by slowing the absorption of carbohydrates

The WHO recommendation for dietary fiber is 27 to 40 grams daily. Meeting this recommendation for the vegetarian athlete is easy, with the abundance of fruits, vegetables, whole grains, and beans consumed regularly. In fact, sometimes vegetarian athletes benefit too much, which is apparent with the "OCCUPIED" signs at the Portosans along the marathon racecourse.

Other drawbacks to getting too much fiber are the chelating or binding effects that cause important minerals such as iron, zinc, calcium, and others (see chapter 7) to be carried out of the body, possibly causing subclinical deficiencies. In addition, fiber-rich carbohydrates may interfere with the body's use of carotene to make vitamin A and may also warrant a higher dietary calcium intake, although vegetarians are less likely to be prone to deficiency (see chapter 1).

Simple Versus Complex for Athletic Performance

Several studies have evaluated the effects of carbohydrates as exercise fuels. Costill and colleagues have compared the effects of complex versus simple carbohydrates during a 48-hour period after glycogen-depleting exercise. Even though complex carbohydrates result in significantly greater muscle glycogen synthesis at 48 hours, the body is less picky for the first 24 hours when it comes to the type of carbs consumed. So go ahead and have a beer and Häagen-Dazs after a big race, but get back into gear with the complex stuff the next day to boost your muscle glycogen levels.

In the long run, complex carbohydrates are best for sports. More nutrient-dense, they provide more B vitamins needed for energy metabolism, iron for oxygen transport, and fiber for a fit digestive tract. All of the athletes' favorite one-pot recipes have adequate complex carbohydrates to meet daily requirements.

The only concern for Ben, Jane, and other runners and athletes is the "bulky excess" problems such as bloating, gas, diarrhea, and dehydration that the additional fibers can cause prior to race time. That full feeling can also limit the amount of calories long-distance athletes consume.

Since endurance athletes rely on complex carbohydrate storage to be at their best before the big event, special food planning must be taken during the "glycogen loading–exercise tapering" period one week prior to a race. Glycogen loading is discussed later in this chapter, while prerace carbo-loading menus are found in chapter 10.

Endurance Performance

For sports that exceed 90 minutes, such as marathon running, swimming, cycling, and triathlon, muscle and liver glycogen is the primary fuel source. Since physical storage of carbohydrates is limited to about 2,400 calories (no more than 2 hours of racing for some sports—see chapter 3), glycogen stores become depleted as the event progresses.

When glycogen stores drop to critically low levels, called glycogen depletion, high-intensity exercise cannot be maintained . . . a.k.a. the athlete "hits the wall"! The athlete can no longer maintain the exercise and needs to quit or dramatically reduce energy output (i.e., speed).

A gradual process over several days can also cause glycogen depletion. The athlete may forget, not prepare, or refuse to consume enough carbohydrates to cover carb expenses used for training. When this happens, the athlete feels flat, heavy, or stale at workouts. To prevent this, approximately 6 to 8 grams of carbohydrate per kilogram of body weight per day is recommended.

This means that the endurance athlete weighing 150 pounds (68 kilograms) needs at least 408 to 544 grams of carbohydrates or up to 700 grams daily. In order to prevent a more serious "glycogen exhaustion," research has shown that athletes who train heavily on successive days must consume about 544 to 680 grams (2,176–2,720 calories), or about 8 to 10 grams of carbohydrate per kilogram of body weight daily. Ultraendurance athletes may require up to 12 to 13 grams of carbohydrates per day to maintain adequate glycogen stores.

Pre-Event Nutrition

Carbohydrate feedings prior to training or competition help restore suboptimal liver glycogen stores. In previous years athletes were told to avoid eating immediately before exercise, specifically high-carbohydrate foods, due to potentially low blood sugar during their event. They were also told to eat 2 to 3 hours before their event in order to avoid GI distress, nausea, and fatigue. These prerace meal myths have since been dispelled. Pre-event nutrition is an industry that has taken on a whole new twist and goes like this.

During exercise, athletes rely upon their existing glycogen and fat stores. Although the pre-exercise meal does not contribute immediate energy, it can provide a source of fuel when an athlete trains for over an hour, or the last meal was consumed 15 hours before the event and glycogen stores are lower.

Research suggests a pre-event carbohydrate intake of 1 to 4 grams of carbohydrate per kilogram of body weight, 1 to 4 hours before the meet.

For example, let's take a 150-pound marathoner:

150 pounds (divided by 2.2) = 68 kilograms

68 kilograms × 1 gram carbohydrate 1 hour before = 68 grams

68 kilograms × 2 grams carbohydrate 2 hours before = 136 grams

68 kilograms × 3 grams carbohydrate 3 hours before = 204 grams

68 kilograms × 4 grams carbohydrate 4 hours before = 272 grams

Prerace foods that are easy to digest, low in fiber, and fortified with vitamins and minerals are best. There are many sport bars, shakes, drinks, and gels available on the market with a variety of sugars, protein, fat, and flavors. An overview of the "final four" for sport performance can be found in this chapter and chapters 6 and 10.

Some of the VSNG athletes' favorite prerace foods and meals are listed below. You can also find Jane's and Ben's favorite pre-competition meals and one-pot dishes at the conclusion of this chapter.

▶ Favorite Pre-Event Meals of ◀ THE VEGETARIAN SPORTS NUTRITION GUIDE Athletes

MOST POPULAR

Pasta with tomato sauce

Plain pasta, bread, salad

Hot cereal

Rice

Whole wheat toast

Pancakes

Beans

Water

OTHER CHOICES

Oatmeal with soy milk and 24 grams soy protein

Large breakfast

Breakfast tarts

Brown rice, kale, banana, blackstrap molasses

Cheerios/Grape Nuts with banana

Mochi

Nut butter

Milk

Juice

Tea

Sport drink

Salmon, vegetables, rice

Stoker Bar, PowerBar, PR Bar, Parillo Bar

Dave Scott's Pre-Event Shake

Fruits

Author's Choice

The night before an event I consume my evening meal before 8:00 P.M. and keep it very bland. I call this "the white diet." The white foods I consume are plain pasta, a few Mrs. T's Pierogies, mashed or baked potato, organic whole wheat or corn tortillas, and a small serving of fat in a dessert or cheese. On the morning of a long race, I will only consume half a sport bar, iced tea, and water.

Often your prerace favorite can change. With unsuccessful racing experiences, your favorite prerace foods can become your worst enemies. Sometimes the company discontinues the brand or formula. This happened with my favorite Ross Exceed sport bars, Joe Weider's Coffee Blast Tiger sport bars, and M&M Mars VO2 Max Bars.

Bar-Hopping

Fortunately, there are new sport bars on store shelves every day. It seems like yesterday when in 1987 Canadian national marathon champion Brian Maxwell and his wife found a unique way to package high-carbohydrate fuel before, during, or after a long run. Their product, called PowerBars, now has a 50% share of the $300-million-dollar yearly worldwide market.

Originally designed for long-distance sports such as cycling, running, hiking, and mountaineering, the market has graduated from supplying energy for serious athletes to a food alternative for busy, health-conscious individuals. The 150- to 300-*plus*-calorie pocket-size meals can be found under the trade names You Are What You Eat, Mountain Lift, Stoker, and Tiger Sport Bars. These bars and others are primarily composed of complex and simple carbohydrate blends with varying amounts of high-quality protein, unsaturated fat, vitamins, minerals, and fiber. The nutritional composition of these bars can be found in the Sport Bar Summary on pages 48 and 49.

The latest ingredients to boost the marketing value of bars are "espresso shot" doses of caffeine, herbs, and antioxidants. PowerBar's Essential, Balance Plus Bar, The Energy Bar Company's sport-specific bars, and the Extreme Ripped Force Bar join the current trend of adding the 3 G's: guarana, ginseng, and ginkgo biloba. Company representatives claim that these herbs are added as potent antioxidants, stress reducers, and energy enhancers.

Other bars are designed primarily for power athletes. These bars also vary in dietary composition and extras added for peak performance. Athletes in power sports tend to prefer lower carbohydrate, high-protein bars while continuing to adhere to low-fat regimens. These high-protein bars include BioX Protein 21 and the Met-Rx High Performance Series Bar.

Another popular bar for bodybuilders and powerlifters is the triple-shot-mocha Extreme Ripped Force Bar, which contains a coffee-cup dose of caffeine (150 mg) and a 300-milligram boost of ma huang. These additives act as physical and mental stimulants and have been shown to act as an ergogenic, so professional athletes need to use caution.

Recently, an American professional athlete was stripped of her Ironman prize money and medal for testing positive for ma huang, called ephedra. This natural herb (see chapter 8) has an amphetamine-like effect on the body and is illegal to use under the IOC guidelines. The bar's nutrition label even includes a warning to individuals with heart, respiratory, and psychiatric problems, a clear discouragement of use for those under 18 years old, and a recommendation to consume no more than one bar daily.

Veteran high-carbohydrate bar users, low-carbohydrate dieters, and others looking for a high-carbohydrate bar alternative for taste, satiation value, and lower sugar content have a good selection of bars to select. Bars such as Balance, Clif, and PR Ironman Bars have even changed the formulation of their forefathers to meet the demand for meal replacements. These bars also tailor to the 40/30/30 eaters, who prefer a higher protein intake of 30% total calories, a higher fat intake of 30%, and fewer total carbohydrates of 40% for athletic performance (see chapter 10).

Popular diets like the Atkins Program have also created new bars for their dieters. GeniSoy is one of the newer bars to jump onto the neutroceuticals bandwagon and keep up with scientific research suggesting the benefits of phytochemicals on health (see chapter 7).

▶ SPORT BAR SUMMARY ▼

Sport Bar	Calories	Protein	Carbohydrates	Sugar	Fat	Saturated Fat	Fiber	Sugar Source	Extras
High Carb/ Fitness Bars									
You Are What You Eat	190*	4*	42*	25	3.0*	1.0	5*	fructose, cane juice, date puree, honey	6–40% RDAs, kosher
Clif Bar	250	10	39	13	5.0	1.0	6	brown rice syrup	up to 150% RDAs
Mountain Lift	210	12	33	20	4.5	3.5	3	corn syrup, maltitol	100% RDAs, 3G's
Twinlab Ultrafuel	230	15	42	15	0	0	2	rice syrup, fruit syrup, maltodextrin	100–420% RDAs
PowerBar Inc.: Original PowerBar	230	10	45	20	2.5	0.5	3	high fructose corn syrup, maltodextrin	35–100% RDAs
Essentials	180	10	28	20	4.0	2.0	3	brown rice syrup	3G's 15–100% RDAs
GeniSoy	210	14	36	18	0	0	1	corn syrup, maltitol	25% RDAs; 100% vitamin E

High Protein Bars

PowerBar, Inc.: PowerPlus	290	24	38	23	5	3.5	2	brown rice syrup, sucrose	glutamine, methionine, BCAAs, 20–35% RDAs 100% RDAs vitamins A,C, E
Met-Rx	340	27	50	29	4	2.0	0	corn syrup, high fructose corn syrup	35–150% RDAs
Protein 21	290	21	40	26	5	3.5	2	fructose, glucose, beet sugar	35% RDAs

Higher Fat and/or Protein Bars

PR Ironman	230	17	25	16	7	2.5	1	high-fructose corn syrup, sucrose	25–50% RDAs
Balance Bar	200	15	22	16	6	4.5	1	high fructose and high maltose corn syrup	up to 100% RDAs (bar dependent)
Parillo Bar	230	14	35	3	6	0	3	rice dextrin, maltodextrin	5 grams medium-chain triglycerides (MCT)

*Dependent on flavor and variety.

Do Sport Bars Work?

Finding a high-carbohydrate, nutritious fuel source that's tolerable when experiencing prerace jitters is always a challenge. Sport bars are ideal for travel and long waiting periods between competitive breaks in sports such as track and field, swimming, diving, dancing, and skating. Although most sports nutritionists would recommend high-carbohydrate whole foods or beverages as prerace meals or snacks, sport bars and sport drinks are a great way to replenish carbohydrates and other nutrients as a snack instead of skipping meals.

The beauty of using the bars is also convenience, packaging, durability, and digestibility of using these bars on the run, while cycling, and under a variety of environmental conditions such as heat, cold, and altitude. Some bars' additives even highlight that aspect. For instance, Mountain Lift provides 100% of antioxidant vitamins A, C, and E for this purpose.

As for the additional fat and protein in the new-generation bars, since most athletes are overly conscientious about fat consumption and are in need of quality protein sources, meeting their needs through the higher-fat, higher-protein choices might help. The 40/30/30 bar may just be what the doctor ordered for fat- and protein-deficient athletes.

Suggestions for selecting a sport bar:

- Try a variety of bars under similar conditions to measure the differences in your performance with different nutrient compositions. Never experiment with a new bar at a competition.

- Drink, drink, drink fluids, preferably water, with the bars.

- Find the best-tasting bar for you. There are hundreds of flavors, textures, and strengths. Check the label for added herbs, supplements, or caffeine that may be illegal to use in your sport.

A chart describing the newest and most popular bars can be found on pages 48–49. Depending on the sport, the time you compete, your size, and hence your carbohydrate needs, many other foods may work better for you. As long as the foods are low in fat, fiber, and lactose and moderate in protein, they should work. The High-Carbohydrate Food and Fluids Table on pages 52–53 will help you select high-carbohydrate foods to energize you before and during competition.

Ben's "Smooth Sailing" Laser Oatmeal

Makes 1 serving

---

2 cups oatmeal

¹/₄ cup soy milk

24 grams soy protein

Prepare the oatmeal according to the package with soy milk and powdered protein mix blended in. "Laser down!"

▶ Nutrients per serving: 490 calories, 66 grams carbohydrates, 39 grams protein, 7 grams fat (unless fat-free soy milk is used)

▶ Dietary composition: 32% protein, 55% carbohydrates, 13% fat

▶ Good source of vitamin E, phosphorus, manganese, and selenium; moderate source of vitamin B_1, magnesium, iron, and zinc

---

For athletes who compete in all-day events such as synchronized swimming, swimming, track and field, basketball, volleyball, or wrestling tournaments, it's difficult to plan pre-event snacks. Therefore, it's best to be prepared with a variety of high-carbohydrate foods and fluids that meet the guidelines suggested above for lasting the entire méet. Some of the spotlight athletes' favorite high-carbohydrate snacks can be found in the table on pages 22–24 in chapter 1.

▶ High-Carbohydrate Foods and Fluids ◀

Food Group/Food	Calories	Carbohydrate (grams)
Fruits		
Apple	81	21
Dried apple, 1 oz	75	21
Applesauce, ½ cup	50	10
Pear	100	25
Grapes, 1 cup	58	16
Banana	120	28
Orange	64	16
Grains		
Bagel	130	30
Bread, whole wheat	60	12
Breadsticks, whole wheat, 3	60	11
Muffin, blueberry	200	29
Cereal, Cheerios, 1 oz	111	20
Corn flakes, 1 oz	100	25
Grape Nuts, 1 oz	101	23
Oatmeal, 1 oz	100	18
Chips, baked, 1 oz (11 potato chips)	110	23
Pancake, buckwheat, 2	143	27
Pretzels, oat bran, 1 oz (20 pretzels)	110	21
Rice, 1 cup	109	22
Saltines, fat-free, 5	60	12
Tortilla, 1 flour	130	23
Waffle, multigrain	250	28
Sweets		
Jell-O, 1 snack pack	70	17
Frozen Fruit Bar, Sunkist	100	25
Rice cakes, Hain Cookie Bits, 17	60	13
Orange Herbal Chews, 27	140	34
Dairy and Dairy Alternatives		
Frozen yogurt, 8 oz	220	42
Dannon Fat Free Yogurt, 6 oz	160	33
Complete Drink, 1 pack	200	33

Food Group/Food	Calories	Carbohydrate (grams)
Balanced Shake	230	37
Stretch Island Fruit Leather	45	12
Other		
Baked potato, small	124	28
Sweet potato, small	117	27
Popcorn, Bearitos, no fat, 1 oz	108	21
Pasta, 2 oz	210	42
Fluids		
Gatorade, 8 oz	50	14
Perform, 8 oz	60	16
Apple juice, 1 cup	111	28

Glycogen Loading for the Millennium

Glycogen loading is a useful technique for delaying glycogen depletion in endurance sports. It allows the athlete to store two to three times the normal amount of glycogen in the muscle. Replenished blood glucose and muscle and liver glycogen stores can fuel exercise for about 2 hours.

The original, more drastic glycogen-loading technique, developed in the late 1960s by Scandinavian researchers, was modified by Dr. Michael Sherman of Ohio State University to prevent some of the side effects such as "heaviness" often reported with the traditional depletion/repletion technique.

To maximize glycogen stores safely, endurance athletes should note the following list.

1. Consume a normal 60 to 75% carbohydrate diet for the training diet.

2. Exercise hard at 70 to 75% aerobic capacity for about 90 minutes to deplete glycogen stores 1 week before the event. Reduce carbohydrate intake to 4 grams per kilogram or 50% of total calories.

3. Following that initial depletion, carbohydrate is reintroduced at about 70% total intake (8–10 grams/kilogram body weight). Training is reduced in time by half to 40 minutes on days 6 and

5 before the event. On days 4 and 3 before competition, exercise is reduced by half again to 20 minutes. Some athletes, however, do well maintaining some level of intensity. They claim it helps them to stay sharp for race day despite the cutback in duration for the taper.

4. The day before competition is rest day. This rest day helps the athlete replenish glycogen stores and prepare mentally for the event. Again, some athletes like a ten- to fifteen-minute stretch or walk around the foreign city or race expo. Either way, the goal is to have a fresh athlete ready and hungry for competition.

The key nutrition thoughts to keep in mind are to maintain a high-carbohydrate diet, but one low in fiber and lactose (milk sugar) and moderate in protein and fat.

Additional Tips for Carbo-Loading

The athlete must be endurance-trained or it won't work. Endurance training increases the activity of glycogen synthetase, the enzyme responsible for glycogen storage. The key is to train extra hard for big events so that when you go to taper, it's actually a taper.

In the final three days, the athlete must reduce training, otherwise glycogen will be used and the procedure will be useless. This is the tough part for most of us, but critical for maximizing glycogen stores and resting and repairing muscle tissue.

The procedure is specific to muscle groups. The exercise to deplete glycogen stores must be the same as the athlete's competitive event. A 2-mile swim to deplete stores for a marathon won't cut it.

Although vegetarian athletes usually consume enough carbohydrates through their normal diet, sometimes traveling can make the task of finding high-carbohydrate vegetarian foods challenging. Adding sport shakes and bars can help, as some of the athletes in this book have discovered. In fact, Jane Welzel consumes only sport drinks and PR Bars prior to competition. I have found that reserving special "race day" foods prepares me to be physically and psychologically pumped up. It's that "race routine". . . same outfit, same shoes, same sequence of events!

Since the program does not improve speed and can add additional water weight, this method is not helpful for shorter distance events and may actually hinder performance. It is not suitable for the local 5K.

▶ Glycogen Loading/Training Regimen ◀

Time	Exercise Duration	Dietary Carbohydrates	Other Tips
Prior to week before competition	endurance trained 1–3 hours or more	8–10 grams /kg/bw	Complex-carb diet, high-fiber, low-fat; minimum of 5 colors per day
Day 7 Depletion day	90 minutes 70–75% max	50% of total calories 4 grams/kg/bw	Include higher-protein meals; maintain high-quality carbs
Day 6 Begin to replenish by reducing exercise	40 minutes	Maintain carbohydrates at 50% total calories	Same
Day 5	Same	Same	Same
Day 4	20 minutes	Increase carbohydrates to 70% total calories or 8–10 grams kg/bw	Decrease fiber and bulk by 5%; reduce dairy intake
Days 3 and 2	Maintain 20 minutes	Maintain carbohydrate intake at 70%	Reduce bulk and fiber; eat small, frequent meals and snacks of 100–500 calories; increase fluids and carbs from sport drinks
Prerace day	Rest/stretch/ pray	Maintain 70% carbs	Less than 10–15 grams fiber, no dairy
Race day	Go for it!	Prerace meal, bar, or snack	As tolerated

Carbohydrate Intake during Endurance Exercise

For events lasting longer than 90 minutes, carbohydrate fuel has been shown to enhance endurance by providing glucose to the muscles when glycogen stores have dropped to low levels. As muscles run out of glycogen, they take sugar from the blood, depleting liver stores. The longer the training session, the more blood sugars are used.

Although blood sugar can be provided by liver glycogen, muscle glycogen cannot because it lacks the enzyme needed to break it down. The result of depletion is dizziness, nausea, confusion, and hypoglycemia. The long-distance athletes in this book can share their tales of "bonking" at races due to glycogen depletion and low blood sugar levels.

> "When they asked me who the president was at mile 18 of the Columbus Marathon and I replied 'Nixon,' they told me the race was over for me."
> —Lisa Dorfman, 1995

I prepared as normal for this marathon, but due to 16°F temperatures, two hours into the race I had used more glycogen than I normally would while training in my 90°F South Florida environment. Therefore, I hit the wall hard and fast!

Several studies have shown that eating 25 to 30 grams of carbohydrates (100–200 calories) every half hour during the race or event may prevent the athlete from having a carbohydrate breakdown. An 8-ounce sport drink or half a package of sport gel can provide this. An abundance of sport gels and fluids can do the trick during long-distance events. Some athletes use bananas, oranges, and sport drinks for long-distance triathlon events. A list of sport gels, drinks, and shakes can be found in chapters 6 and 10.

Carbohydrate Intake after Exercise

The best time to replenish glycogen stores after strenuous training is immediately after exercise. At this time, blood flow is much greater to the muscles and therefore takes more glucose to the muscle. Also, the muscle cells are more sensitive to insulin, which promotes glycogen synthesis.

Waiting too long after a race to eat can be detrimental to glycogen storage replacement and recovery. Delaying a postrace meal by 2 hours, research shows, results in a reduction in muscle glycogen synthesis of up to 66%. By 4 hours, muscle glycogen synthesis can be 45% slower than when food is consumed immediately after exercise.

Postrace carbohydrate recommendations are about 2 grams of simple carbohydrates per kilogram of body weight immediately after the race. To help replenish muscle glycogen stores, about 100 grams carbohydrate (400 calories) every 2 hours is recommended until the next meal. The total carbohydrate intake for the next 24 hours should be about 9 to 10 grams per kilogram of body weight. For lightweight Lisa at 104 pounds, this means an intake of 94 to 100 grams of carbohydrates after crossing the race line and a minimum of 468 grams of carbohydrates during the first 24 hours after the event.

Since rejoicing after the marathon or long-distance triathlon is the first thing on my mind, thinking about consuming food is a challenge. Fortunately, many of my favorite races offer foods and drinks that are easy to tolerate. At Grandma's Marathon in Duluth, Minnesota, XLR 8 high-carb drinks have been served. At another favorite, Big Sur Marathon in California, juice, frozen fruit pops, and sport drinks hit the spot after conquering the famous Hurricane Point. In abnormally cold and wet weather for the Marine Corps Marathon the year Oprah made her marathon debut, hot chocolate, cookies, soup, and crackers were available at the finish. Disney World's Mickey Mouse greets you with a smile and a high-carb buffet after that world-class event.

Some athletes prefer to wait in the beer line. This is a viable option, since beer replaces carbohydrates and helps the athlete relax or celebrate the finish. The pros and cons of alcohol and sports performance are discussed in chapter 6.

After I've showered and my belly is ready to rumble to the dinner table, some of my favorite recovery recipes include Hanners' Vegetarian Chili, Rice and Red Beans, and my Bean Taco Pie on pages 58, 59, and 60 respectively. I generally continue to consume water and other fluids throughout the night.

Hanners' Vegetarian Chili

Makes 4 servings

½ onion, diced

1 red and 1 green pepper, diced

2 tsp olive oil

2 jalapeños, diced (optional)

3 cups tomatoes, chopped

1 cup vegetable juice (V8 is ok)

2 tbs cumin

2 tbs chili powder

salt and pepper

1 bay leaf

¾ cup texturized vegetable protein (TVP)

2 cups vegetable stock

Sauté diced vegetables in olive oil. Add tomatoes and stew for 5 minutes. Add V8 juice and continue to simmer. Add seasonings and bay leaf. Add TVP and allow to absorb tomato flavor before adding stock. Simmer on low for 30 minutes.

▶ Nutrients per serving: 333 calories, 24 grams protein, 46 grams carbohydrates, 8 grams fat, 3.5 grams monounsaturated fat, 1 gram linoleic fat, 19 grams sugar, 10 grams fiber

▶ Dietary composition: 27% protein, 51% carbohydrates, 22% fat

▶ VSNG food servings: 2.5 cups vegetables, 1.5 proteins, 1 fat

▶ Good source of vitamin A, C, K, folate, potassium, iron; moderate source of vitamin B_2, B_6, E, copper, manganese

Hanners' Rice and Red Beans

Makes 2 servings

––––––––

$^1/_2$ cup kidney beans

$^1/_2$ cup pinto beans

vegetable stock as needed

2 tsp cumin

$^1/_2$ tsp cayenne

1 cup long-grain brown rice

$^1/_2$ onion, diced

salt and pepper

––––––––

Soak beans overnight. Rinse well. Bring beans to a boil in seasoned vegetable stock. Add the onions and spices. Reduce to a simmer and cook until tender. Using bean broth, add rice and cook until dish becomes one. Season to taste with salt and pepper.

▶ Nutrients per serving: 466 calories, 15 grams protein, 93 grams carbohydrates, 4 grams fat, 1 gram monounsaturated fat, 1 gram linoleic fat, 5 grams fiber

▶ Dietary composition: 13% protein, 80% carbohydrates, 7% fat

▶ VSNG food servings: 6 grains, $^1/_2$ protein

Lisa's Bean Taco Pie

Makes 1 serving

———

flour tortilla, flavored or organic whole wheat if possible
$^1/_4$ cup refried beans (Shari's or Fantastic Foods)
$^1/_4$ cup Hanners' Vegetarian Chili (see page 58)
or Health Valley canned organic chili
1 oz grated soy cheese
$^1/_4$ cup frozen corn

———

Layer in baking tin, beginning with $^1/_4$ large tortilla, then refried beans, corn, chili, and cheese. Repeat twice and top with tortilla quarter and grated soy cheese. Bake for approximately 15–20 minutes at 325 degrees F.

▶ Nutrients per serving; 255 calories, 17 grams protein, 41 grams carbohydrates, 3 grams fat
▶ Dietary composition: 26% protein, 63% carbohydrates, 11% fat
▶ VSNG food servings: 1 protein, 2 grains, $^1/_2$ vegetable
▶ Moderate source of vitamin C, folate, and iron

Food fitness note: Adapted from Wild Oats Food Market and Gardner's Market (Miami)

Postevent Tips

Another factor to consider for postrace meals is the transit time of food through the GI tract. Research suggests that colder-than-body-temperature, low-fat, and acidic foods leave the stomach quicker and are absorbed by the system sooner. That means that cool oranges, citrus juices, or pops may work best for athletes sensitive to gut distress after racing.

Warmer, high-fat, high-fiber, and higher calorie (nutrient-dense) foods and fluids stay in the system longer. These foods are especially soothing to the cold and "battered" athlete.

Carbohydrate Prescription (Rx)

There are a few ways to calculate the total amount of carbohydrates you need daily. In order to figure out the amount of grams of carbohydrates needed daily, follow these steps:

1. Take the amount of calories you need to consume daily to maintain your desired weight.

2. Multiply this number by 60 to 75%, or see the carbohydrate chart for a specific carbohydrate recommendation.

3. Take your total carbohydrate intake gram recommendation and multiply this by 10% to get your daily recommendation of simple carbohydrate grams.

4. Take the simple carbohydrate grams and divide by four to get the amount of teaspoons of simple sugars. This is an eye-opener.

5. Check your food labels and the carbohydrate gram lists in this book to calculate the amount you can get from the plant-based foods you consume or desire to consume daily.

High Carbs Versus High-Fat Diets for Performance

Although this issue is addressed in chapter 5 and other chapters, I hope that after reading this chapter and the book, you are convinced that there is no question that high-carbohydrate diets are critical to sports performance. Vegetarian diets are perhaps part of the reason that the Olympic and world-class athletes in this book and elsewhere excel at their sports.

If you have concerns about the effect of carbohydrates on your program or performance, ask yourself the following:

▶ Where do you get most of your carbohydrate, simple or complex, foods?

▶ Do you get enough variety, or do you get into carbohydrate "jags," eating the same foods every day like a small toddler? If

Calculating Your Carbohydrate Rx

1. For example, on 2,000 calories, you need 1,200–1,500 calories of carbohydrates.

2. Divide these calorie numbers by 4 to get carbohydrate grams, which are 300 to 375 grams of carbohydrates.

3. Take total carbohydrate grams and multiply by 10% (.10) to get the grams of simple sugars. This is about 30 to 37 grams of sugar daily.

4. Take your sugar grams and divide by 4 to get teaspoons of sugar recommended daily. This comes to about 7$\frac{1}{2}$ to 9 teaspoons daily.

5. Check your food labels. If your sport bar contains 28 grams of sugar, you have eaten practically your entire suggested total daily sugar intake. Check all food labels, natural, organic, healthy, or not. Sometime the "healthy" food has more sugar. For instance, my daughter's 100% natural, no-added-sugar juice box for school has 30 grams of sugar (7.5 teaspoons), while a serving of Gatorade has 18 grams (4.5 teaspoons). Surprised? Don't be. Check those labels.

6. Then make a decision to make better choices, lower in sugar, to feel and perform better. Even with sport bars, there are some on the market with less simple sugar. Gary's favorite Parillo Bars only contain 3 grams of sugar, Clif Bar has just 13 grams (3 tsp), and Twinlab Ultrafuel has 15 grams (4 tsp). Check out the sport bar table in this chapter to see how much your favorite bar has. Make a choice.

you eat bagels and pasta daily, at least vary the types. Many bagel stores offer plain, cinnamon raisin, poppy, sesame, and more. Pasta comes in whole wheat, quinoa, corn, spinach, and tomato flavors. By varying your choices, you are bound to get more of the missing vitamins, minerals, fiber, phytochemicals, and other unknown beneficial compounds whose deficiencies are hindering your performance.

▶ Are you getting enough or too much carbohydrates? Check the charts and do your calculations. Too little can leave you depleted; too much can make you bloated, heavy, and fatter than desired.

▶ How much of your food is fresh, organic, and unprocessed? Chemicals and lack of fiber will affect how you feel (and function!).

▶ How many teaspoons of sugar do you eat? Even though you are consuming enough carbohydrates, perhaps you are getting too much from simple sugars. Simple sugars will rob your body of vitamins and minerals that you can get from healthier choices.

▶ When is the best time to consume your carbohydrates? Since exercise may diminish appetites, athletes may wait until after their last workout to eat and overdo it. Limiting calories to 250–500 calories at a meal instead of 1,000-plus will keep you leaner, especially if you're female and older. Eating too many carbohydrates at one time may cause you to feel too full, bloated, or sleepy. Not only do carbohydrates hold about 3 grams of water for every gram consumed but a brain chemical called serotonin is produced in large quantities after high-carbohydrate meals. This can make you sleepy.

How can you use this to your advantage? Instead of eating a bowl of pasta and basket of rolls for lunch, consume your largest carbohydrate meal in the evening, 2 hours before bedtime. The meal will help you to sleep and will fuel you for the morning workout.

Welzel's Marathon CousCous

Makes 2 servings

---

2 cups cooked couscous or rice

1 cup frozen corn

1 cup frozen green beans

1 cup frozen carrots

1 cup frozen broccoli

½ cup great northern beans

1 tsp curry paste*

about 8 oz seitan

Mix, serve, run.

▶ Nutrients per serving: 470 calories, 25 grams protein, 90 grams carbohydrates, 5 grams fat, 10 grams sugar, 18 grams fiber

▶ Dietary composition: 19% protein, 71% carbohydrates, 9% fat

▶ VSNG food servings: 3 vegetables, 4 grains, 1 fat

▶ Good source of vitamin A, B_6, C, K, folate, potassium, selenium, manganese; moderate source of vitamin B_1, B_2, B_3, pantothenic acid, phosphorus, magnesium, iron, zinc, and copper

*Food fitness note: Pataks makes great curry paste in mild or extra-hot.

Jane Welzel

1990 U.S. National Marathon Champion,
2:33 marathoner

Spotlight Athlete

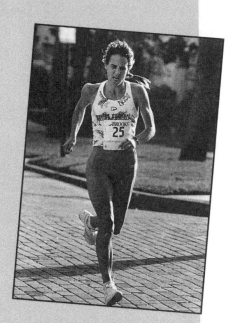

Age: 43

23 years lacto-ovo-vegetarian

Reason for becoming vegetarian:
"We raised some of our own
animals and I couldn't make
that leap from pet to dinner."

Advantages of being vegetarian:
"Healthy diet, foods easy to
digest between workouts."

Challenges to being vegetarian:
"When we go to races in
some parts of the country, it
is hard to get vegetarian protein sources and the type of
foods I prefer. So I travel with protein powder and PR Bars in
case. I must take iron supplements because I am anemic."

Alcohol: merlot wine five days a week and beer once a week

Supplements: vitamin C, iron, multivitamin (PR Bars, protein
powder, various sport drinks—only for marathons and long
runs)

Favorite prerace meal: "In the morning before a race I have one
half to one PR Bar. The night before I usually have a pasta
dish."

Favorite snacks: tofu pops, tofu snacks, candy, tortilla chips,
crackers, and hummus (in the summer, popsicles)

Favorite one-pot meal: Welzel's Marathon CousCous
(page 64)

Wurzel and Mathews' Marathon Prerace Pasta Blaster

Makes 1 serving

———

8 oz fresh pasta
$\frac{1}{2}$ cup red sauce (try Enrico's)

———

Prepare fresh pasta. Add $\frac{1}{2}$ cup of warmed red sauce over cooked pasta.

▶ Nutrients per serving: 344 calories, 14 grams protein, 65 grams carbohydrates, 2 grams fat, 4 grams fiber

▶ Dietary composition: 16% protein, 78% carbohydrates, 6% fat

▶ VSNG food servings: 1 vegetable, 4 grains

▶ Moderate source of vitamin B_1, B_2, iron

Ben Mathews

*Masters marathon sensation
and ultramarathoner*

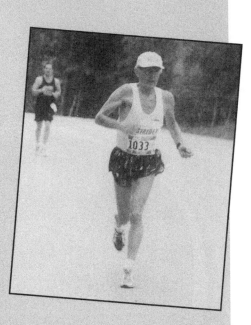

▷ *Age:* 60

▷ 7 years macrobiotic
vegetarian

▷ *Reason for becoming
vegetarian:* "Health,
improve performance,
control weight,
strengthen the
immune system."

▷ *Advantages of being
vegetarian:* "Weight
control, source of
good nutrition."

▷ *Challenges to being vegetarian:*
"Finding the right food to eat when traveling away from
home."

▷ *Alcohol:* none

▷ *Supplements:* no supplements or medications

▷ *Favorite prerace meal:* pasta with red sauce

▷ *Favorite snacks:* raisins and bananas

▷ *Favorite one-pot meal:* Mathews' Marathon BBQ Tempeh (see
page 84)

4

Protein: The Fitness Powerhouse

VEGETARIANISM draws all kinds of people together, from all walks of life, professions, and experiences. Art Still is a phenomenal athlete and human being whom I've grown to respect and adore since the first time I interviewed him for this book. His gracious vegetarian wife, Liz, became my e-mail pal when I was writing this book.

As a two-time MVP and four-time Pro Bowl player, Art is an accomplished and respected athlete. As a father to nine vegetarian children, four of whom are adopted, his life with Liz on a fifteen-acre farm in western New York encompassed the peaceful life this 6-foot-7-inch, 255-pound vegetarian former defensive end chose to offer his family. (Art has since relocated to Kansas.) As I said before, vegetarianism goes far beyond eating carrot sticks and granola bars.

Currently 43 years old, Art became a semivegetarian 19 years ago, and was a practicing vegan for 5 years of that time. His reason for becoming vegetarian was to lead a healthier lifestyle and get more energy and endurance. Can you hear the guys at the training table now! In addition to having more energy and endurance, Art found it a great way to keep his weight and body fat down. However, he often found it challenging to find certain foods while traveling and maintain the right proportion of foods for muscle growth.

The Science of Proteins

If a 255-pound, 6-foot-7-inch Hall of Fame defensive end can get enough protein to build strength and endurance, you can too! Protein makes up the second-largest percentage of material in the body, after water. The average body stores about 11 grams of protein, 40% residing in muscle. There are as many as 10,000 different proteins in every human cell that program life's processes. Without protein, life (and sport) would not exist.

Even though protein is not a major source of energy for sport (except in special circumstances), protein is critical to the health of the athlete. The box below shows the many ways proteins work in the human body.

▶ Functions of Protein ◀

Structure	maintains skin, hair, muscle, bones, and teeth
Growth and maintenance	builds and repairs body tissues
Enzymes and hormones	regulates the body's processes in digestion and metabolism
Immune system	builds antibodies to protect the body from infection
Hemoglobin and myoglobin	forms blood proteins involved in energy transport to the muscles
Muscle proteins	makes muscle-contracting proteins called actin and myosin
pH	maintains a delicate balance for chemical reactions such as digestion to function properly
A vehicle	transports other nutrients around the body, for example, lipoproteins for fat

Protein differs from carbohydrates and fats because it contains nitrogen in its structure. This nitrogen atom gives the name "amino" (nitrogen-containing) to the amino acids of which protein is made. Nitrogen balance is used as a measurement to evaluate protein needs.

Nitrogen Balance Studies

Nitrogen balance studies are a difficult and expensive way to compare the difference between all sources of protein intake (16% of which is nitrogen) and nitrogen loss through urine, feces, sweat, etc. This method is sensitive to changes in total calorie intake, energy output, percentage of protein, fats, and carbohydrates consumed, and time spent in measuring a true balance.

A positive balance occurs during growth periods, pregnancy, bodybuilding, tissue growth replenishment, or recovery from a deficiency. A negative balance is a result of deficiency of one or more essential amino acids, fasting, starvation, burns, injury, trauma, infections, and fever. Skin losses account for 5 to 8 mg of nitrogen per kilogram of body weight per day; feces, 12 mg; and urine, 37 mg, for a total of 54 mg nitrogen (approximately .45 grams protein/kg/day).

While carbohydrates have repeating identical units in their structure, all amino acid chains are different. Variations in the number, proportion, and order of amino acids allow for an infinite number of protein structures. This is partially how protein gives us all a uniqueness that cannot be replicated. The sequence of amino acids is specified by heredity and creates our own individual structure and mental and physical characteristics. The likelihood of being an outstanding athlete depends more on your ancestors than on your training—even if they didn't participate in sports.

Amino Acids

Regardless of the food source, proteins are made of amino acids. Requirements for protein actually reflect amino acid needs. Of the twenty amino acids found in foods, nine cannot be made by the body and are called essential. The essential and nonessential amino acids are listed below.

▶ Essential and Nonessential Amino Acids ◀

ESSENTIAL	NONESSENTIAL
Histidine*	Alanine
Isoleucine	Arginine
Leucine	Asparagine
Lysine	Aspartic Acid
Methionine	Cysteine
Phenylalanine	Glutamic Acid
Threonine	Glutamine
Tryptophan	Glycine
Valine	Proline
	Serine
	Tyrosine

*Essential for infants and children

If your diet is deficient in one or more amino acids, the functions of protein cannot continue in the body. That means that you'll still be able to play your favorite sport, but you're more likely to get sick, lose your hair, have a poor complexion, and lose stamina and energy if you're deficient in the essential nine.

Animal products contain all essential amino acids, while plant proteins may be limiting in one or two. Most people don't even realize that grains, vegetables, soy, and nuts contain protein. That's why the first question a meat eater asks when meeting a vegetarian is, "How do you get enough protein?" A list of the "limiting" essential amino acids in plant-based foods can be found on pages 73–74.

Contrary to popular belief and concerns from the medical community and the public at large, vegetarians can easily get enough protein in their diets. Athletes who are semi- or lacto-ovo-vegetarian usually consume enough because of the high-protein density of milk, dairy, eggs, chicken, and fish. On the average, vegetarian diets contain 12.5% of energy from protein. The VSNG athletes average a higher protein level of 20% (99 grams) of total calories. As food options become more limited, it generally becomes more challenging to get enough protein. However, even strict vegans have been shown to meet their protein needs.

On the average, vegans consume approximately 11% total calories from protein. By eating enough complementary "limiting" protein sources over the course of the day, protein requirements can be easily met. In fact, the VSNG vegan athletes reported an intake of about 17% (73 grams) of their total calorie intake from protein, demonstrating that they are hardly deficiency candidates, while the more liberal lacto-ovo VSNG athletes averaged about 15% protein (61 grams) daily.

Since Art, Jane, and other athletes such as Ben, Craig, and Erika often compete in small towns and abroad, nonanimal protein sources are difficult to find. High-protein, portable vegetarian snacks and meals are listed in this chapter and chapter 1, while high-protein meals can be found in chapter 10.

▶ Limiting Essential Amino Acids in Plant-Based Foods ◀

FOOD	AMINO ACID
Grains	
Maize or corn	lysine, tryptophan
Millet	lysine, threonine
Oats	lysine, threonine
Wheat	lysine, threonine
Rice	lysine, threonine
Legumes	
Beans—immature	methionine, isoleucine
Beans—mature	methionine, valine
Peanuts	lysine, threonine

FOOD	AMINO ACID
Nuts and oil seeds	
Coconut	lysine, threonine
Soybeans	methionine
Sesame and sunflower seeds	lysine
Peanuts	lysine, methionine, threonine
Cottonseed	lysine
Vegetables	
Green leafy	methionine
Peas	methionine, tryptophan
Other	
Gelatin	methionine, lysine, tryptophan
Yeast	phenylalanine

A quick look at the above list shows some natural complementary combinations of foods such as rice and beans, pasta with peas and greens, and nut butter on crackers. Other quick combinations, found later in the book, are "one-pot" complementary, peak-performance favorites including Abate's Deca-Minestrone (page 75) and Hanners' Fava Bean Hummus with crackers or toasted whole wheat pita (page 76).

One of my favorite high-protein afternoon snack combos is tofu-based cheese (Soya Kaas or Vegan Rella), organic whole wheat tortillas, baked chips, rice or wheat crackers, and an apple. Other athletes enjoy Mexican meals with beans, tortillas, vegetables, and cheese (see Heath's Skating Mexican Fiesta Meal, chapter 5, page 95).

Measuring Protein Quality

There are many ways to measure the quality of food proteins. Three methods are the Amino Acid Score, Protein Efficiency Ratio, and the most useful, *Protein Digestibility–Corrected Amino Acid Score (PDCAAS)*. This is the most important measurement of the amount geared toward supporting the maintenance of body tissues in adults. It is used to establish the protein values listed on food labels.

Abate's Deca-Minestrone

Makes 4 servings

2 cloves garlic

1 small onion, chopped

3 stalks celery

8 cups vegetable stock

basil

1 28-oz can tomatoes, chef's cut*

$\frac{1}{2}$ bag mixed frozen veggies, 16 oz.

1 15 oz can red kidney beans*

1 15 oz can white kidney beans*

5 oz penne pasta

Sauté the garlic, onion, and celery in a medium to large stewpot. Add the vegetable stock and basil. Toss in the tomatoes, veggies, and beans. Cook on medium heat for 2 to 5 minutes. Add the pasta and simmer for 15 minutes. Add a dash of salt and pepper to taste. Serve with fresh parmesan cheese. Mangia!

▶ Nutrients per serving: 335 calories, 19 grams protein, 65 grams carbohydrate, 2 grams fat

▶ Dietary composition: 21% protein, 74% carbohydrate, 5% fat

▶ VSNG food servings: 2 cups vegetables, 3 grains

▶ Good source of vitamin A, B_6, C, potassium, iron; moderate source of folate, pantothenic acid, phosphorus, copper

*Food fitness note: choose organic canned beans; buy fresh tomatoes when possible

---
▼

Hanners' Fava Bean Hummus

Makes 5 servings

———

2 cups shelled fava beans

zest of 1 lemon

3 cloves garlic

1 tsp olive oil

salt and pepper to taste

———

Purée all the ingredients in a food processor or blender until smooth.

▶ Nutrients per serving: 97 calories, 4 grams protein, 17 grams carbohydrate, 1 gram fat, 2 grams sugar, 5 grams fiber

▶ Dietary composition: 19% protein, 70% carbohydrates, 10% fat

▶ VSNG food servings: 1 grain

▶ Source of vitamin C, potassium, and manganese

In addition to the food's amino acid balance, the digestibility of protein is a critical element in evaluating protein sources. Egg whites hold the highest PDCAAS score, of 100. Milk protein (casein) also has a 100. Perhaps that's why lacto-ovo-vegetarians often have an easier time meeting their complete protein needs.

Soybeans are the only plant-based food that meet an ideal profile. Roots and tubers have half the amount of nitrogen of soybeans and primarily the nonessential amino acids glutamine and asparagine. Seeds and grains have 95% or more of their protein as nitrogen.

Vegetarian menus that have the highest PDCAAS foods benefit the athlete by providing the most biologically available nonanimal proteins for peak performance. Recipes including these nutrient-packed foods can be found throughout the book. Hanners' Fava Bean Hummus is a recipe with a high PDCAAS score.

One of my personal ovo-vegetarian favorites is Eggology scrambled egg whites mixed with green peas (see page 77). Topping my list of vegan-based high-PDCAAS food is Bean Taco Pie (chapter 3, page 60), prepared with beans, tortillas, and soy cheese. A listing of nonanimal protein PDCAAS food scores appears on page 78.

Lisa's Scrambled Whites and Greens

Makes 1 serving

---

vegetable oil spray
2 servings Eggology egg whites, according to package
½ cup frozen green peas
sea salt

Spray frying pan with Pam-type spray. Heat pan. Blend egg whites and peas and throw in pan. Cook until whites are coagulated (white, not clear). Salt to taste. Voila!

▶ Nutrients per serving: 183 calories, 30 grams protein, 13 grams carbohydrates, 0 fat

▶ Dietary composition: 68% protein, 30% carbohydrates, less than 1% fat

▶ VSNG food servings: 2 protein, 1.5 grains

▶ Good source of vitamin K

▶ Comments: Great meal after hard workout. Can double or triple recipe for more calories and/or protein.

Variation Scrambled Whites with Spinach and Mushrooms

Makes 1 serving

---

4 servings Eggology egg whites, according to package
½ cup fresh spinach
½ cup mushrooms (maitake if you can find them)
vegetable oil spray

Same procedure. Chow!

▶ Nutrients per serving: 255 calories, 54 grams protein, 6 grams carbohydrates, 0 fat

▶ Dietary composition: 88% protein, 11% carbohydrates, 1% fat

▶ VSNG food servings: 4 protein, 1 cup vegetables

▶ Good source of vitamin K, moderate source of folate

▶ Protein Digestibility–Corrected Amino Acid ◀ Scores (PDCAAS) of Selected Nonanimal Proteins

Food	PDCAAS %*
Soybeans	94
Whole wheat-pea flour**	82
Chickpeas	69
Kidney beans	68
Peas	67
Pinto beans	61
Rolled oats	57
Black beans	53
Lentils	52
Peanut meal	52
Whole wheat	40
Wheat protein (gluten)	25

*Compared with egg white and milk protein (casein)
**An example of mutual supplementation
Adapted from Hamilton and Whitney's *Nutrition Concepts and Controversies,* 1994.

Protein Requirements for Athletes

The average American consumes about 80 to 125 grams of protein per day. Since 1900, the proportion from animal protein has doubled to 70%. Athletes have been shown to consume nearly double the RDA for protein. In a 1994 study, athletes' protein intakes accounted for 13 to 17% of total energy intake. The protein intake of the vegetarian athletes in this book is 13 to 35%. In 1985, the World Health Organization (WHO) and others developed guidelines for protein requirements that have been accepted by the United States and Canada. The range of calories from protein recommended by the WHO and others is 10 to 15% total calories.

In the 1970s and 1980s, new techniques for estimating protein needs for endurance and strength athletes have shown that active individuals may benefit from 50 to 125% more protein than the current RDA. The factors affecting dietary protein needs are

1. total calorie intake

2. degree of training

3. intensity of training

The most important factor affecting protein requirement is calorie intake. Protein requirements decrease as food intake increases. When food intake is restricted to reach a specific body weight, protein needs may be elevated. This may be especially true for Laser sailor Ben and equestrian show-jumper Debbie.

Anaerobic exercise such as track repeats, cycling crits, and Laser sailing races may cause a greater increase in protein breakdown. Research has shown that protein losses increase with heavy training or during the onset of a new strenuous training program, such as coming back from off-season for the ironman athlete or marathon runner.

Also, there are greater losses up to ten days after a long-distance event like the ironman. These losses can repress the immune system, hinder muscle recovery, and affect other structural and functional needs when protein and/or calorie needs are not adequately met. However, protein deficiency is not usually a risk in industrialized countries or with vegetarian athletes. According to protein experts, protein intakes for athletes of 12 to 15% of total calories on an adequate diet have been found to avoid deficiencies.

Branched chain amino acids (BCAAs) are used preferentially during exercise over others. These BCAAs include the essential amino acids leucine, isoleucine, and valine. Research on traumatic stress and injury patients has shown increased protein breakdown, especially of the BCAAs in muscle. Athletes often use BCAAs as a supplement to prevent muscle breakdown (see chapter 4). BCAAs are also included in the formulas of some sport drinks and lifestyle beverages (see chapter 6).

In addition to BCAA losses, stress also increases glucose production from noncarbohydrate sources and depresses protein synthesis. Hence, if athletes maintain low glycogen stores, the use of protein doubles.

The Ideal Protein Prescription

There is no "ideal" protein prescription since fluctuations in training, conditions, and life will affect daily needs. A close estimate can be calculated by the following formulas and keeping the following in mind.

Relative to body weight, athletes' protein intakes appear to be above 1.5 grams/kilogram/day, while intakes above 2 grams per kilogram per day are common. This is higher than the recommendations in the ideal protein prescription below.

Take the number of grams of protein you calculate and listen to your body carefully. Add additional protein when beginning a new program or during times of intense strength and endurance training. Take away protein when your muscles feel too heavy.

If you calculate a number based on your training, weight, and general guidelines and you find you're feeling heavy or dehydrated, perhaps you are consuming too much protein. If you calculate too low a number for your needs, you will begin to feel run-down, lose hair, break out in pimples, or get sick easily.

To figure out your daily recommended protein intake:

1. Find your body weight.

2. Convert your weight in pounds to kilograms by taking pounds and dividing by 2.2.

3. Multiply the following numbers by your kilogram number to figure out your daily protein needs.

Strength Athletes	Kilograms × 1.2 – 1.7
Endurance Athletes	Kilograms × 1.2 – 1.4
Early Training	Kilograms × 2
Average Active Adult	RDA – kilograms × 0.8 grams

This means that Art, at 255 pounds (116 kilograms), might need a range of 139 grams to 232 grams daily to meet his needs as a defensive end. Each ounce of animal protein is approximately 7 grams.

Other protein values can be found in the chart at the end of this chapter.

Protein Needs for Bodybuilding

Although we don't know exactly how much muscle tissue an athlete can build in a given time period, an educated "guesstimate" has been made by experts. At best, an adult in weight training may be able to add one kilogram of muscle per week. Since muscle is about 20% protein, the following formula can be used to calculate the amount of protein needed (above the minimal requirements) to add this extra kilogram of muscle:

1. Since muscle is 20% protein, to build 1 kilogram (2.2 pounds), take 0.2 kg muscle, which requires 200 extra grams of protein per week.

2. Take 200 grams and divide by 7 days, and you get about 28 grams of protein per day in addition to your daily needs.

3. Now you can take your Protein Rx to the VSNG food lists and find the amount of protein food servings appropriate to meet your needs.

Weight training itself may actually improve the efficiency of protein utilization.

Examples of high-protein plant-based foods and their protein contents are listed below. Art's favorite stir-fry recipe can be made with additional protein sources such as Eggology egg whites, tofu, tempeh, or seitan. See page 82 for Still's "Defensive" Stir-Fry.

▶ High-Protein Vegetarian Food Choices* ◀

Food/Amount	Protein (grams)	Calories	Fat (grams)
Egg, 1 large	7	88	6.0
Egg whites, Eggology, 1/2 cup	13	61	0
Lactaid Fat Free Milk, 1 cup	9	90	0
Cottage cheese, fat-free, 1/2 cup	13	80	0
Beans, 1/2 cup	7	100	0
Tofu, Mori-Nu Lite, 3 oz	6	35	0.5

Food/Amount	Protein (grams)	Calories	Fat (grams)
Yogurt, 1 cup organic	10	180	0
Mozzarella cheese, soy-based, 2 oz	14	60	0
Soy beverage, fat-free, 1 cup	3	90	0
Pasta, 3/4 cup, uncooked	7	210	1.0
Polenta, Fantastic Foods, 3/8 cup	8	260	5.0
Texturized vegetable protein, 1/4 cup	12	80	0
PowerBar	10	230	2.0
Power Chips	10	162	2.0
PowerBar's Protein Plus Bar	24	290	5.0

Note: Other high-protein snacks can be found in the VSNG food lists in chapter 9.

Still's "Defensive" Stir-Fry

Makes 1 serving

———

1 cup cabbage

1 cup shredded carrots

1 cup broccoli florettes

1 cup mushrooms

1 cup mung bean sprouts

1 red pepper, diced

2 tsp peanut oil

———

Fry it up! Serve. Hike!

▶ Nutrients per serving: 214 calories, 14 grams protein, 38 grams carbohydrates, 5 grams fat, 1 gram monounsaturated fat, 1 gram linoleic fat, 19 grams sugar, 13 grams fiber

▶ Dietary composition: 22% protein, 62% carbohydrates, 17% fat

▶ VSNG food servings: 4 cups vegetables, 1/2 fat

▶ Good sources of vitamin A, C, K, folate, pantothenic acid, potassium; moderate source of vitamin B_1, B_2, B_3, B_6, phosphorus, magnesium, iron, copper, manganese

Spotlight Athlete

Art Still

*Former Buffalo Bills and Kansas City
Chiefs MVP defensive end;
Kansas City Chiefs Hall of Fame*

Married, 9 children (4 adopted)

Age: 43

19 years semivegetarian
  (vegan for 5 years)

Reason for becoming vegetarian:
  "Healthier lifestyle, energy,
  and endurance."

Advantages of being vegetarian:
  "More energy and
  endurance. Great way to
  keep weight and body fat
  down."

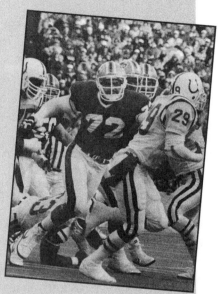

Challenges to being vegetarian: "Availability of
  certain foods while traveling. Also keeping
  right proportion of foods for muscle growth."

Supplements: multivitamin, Nutri-Rx with creatine

Favorite pregame meal: "Plenty of water, raw fruits, and maybe
  pancakes."

Favorite snacks: popcorn, chips, and salsa

Favorite one-pot meal: Still's "Defensive" Stir-Fry (see page 82)

Mathews' Marathon BBQ Tempeh

Makes 2 servings

8 oz block tempeh
1 scallion, chopped
$\frac{1}{4}$ cup shoyu or soy sauce
1 mushroom, sliced
$\frac{1}{4}$ cup snow peas
2 tbs brown rice syrup
1 tsp stone-ground mustard
1 clove garlic, minced
1 tsp onion, minced

Cut the tempeh into thin slices. Marinate in soy sauce, garlic, onion, and seasoning at least 2 hours or overnight. Brown on both sides in lightly oiled skillet. Garnish with chopped scallion. Top with mushrooms and snow peas. Serve with rice or noodles.

▶ Nutrients per serving: 246 calories, 19 grams protein, 29 grams carbohydrates, 7 grams fat, 1.5 grams mono-unsaturated fats, 3 grams linoleic fat

▶ Dietary composition: 30% protein, 46% carbohydrates, 23% fat

▶ VSNG food servings: 1.5 grains, 1 fat

5

Fat Talk

TWO ATHLETES who spend long periods of time training and excelling at their unique sports are Gary Gromet, double ironman triathlete and marathon runner, and Jonathan Didonato, Guinness record-holding long-distance swimmer.

Gary, a pesco-vegetarian for 13 years who took up running in 1986 and the triathlon in 1989, chose vegetarianism to be healthier and participate at an optimum level. He speaks from experience. At 54 and as finisher of two double ironmans, five ironmans, and numerous half-ironmans, cycling races, and marathons, he knows the value of food and fats for the long haul. He finds no challenges to being a vegetarian, even on the road. Gary is always prepared. I had the experience of traveling with him and his wife to the 100th Boston Marathon. One whole suitcase was devoted to healthy foods, soups, breads, and snacks.

Jonathan Didonato, a semivegetarian for 19 years, and his vegetarian identical twin, James, are in the *Guinness Book of Records* as the first brothers to complete the longest butterfly stroke swim, from the Bahamas to Florida. Jonathan chose vegetarianism for stamina and to excel at his sport. As a result, he says he is "indefatigable."

While Jonathan takes no medication, drinks no alcohol, and only supplements with sport shakes and bee pollen, Gary indulges in a glass of Cabernet Sauvignon four times a week and takes a multitude of supplements, including Vitamin E, C, CoQ10, creatine, carnitine, melatonin, grapeseed, ginseng, ginkgo, and biloba. Gary's financial advantage in obtaining these supplements is being in the business. (Gary owns his own health food store in Homestead, Florida.) The value of his pills will be discussed in chapter 8.

Both men enjoy their favorite one-pot recipes, which include fat from olive oil and tofu. How do these fat sources differ? What value do they have to their training programs and health? How much fat should an athlete include in his daily diet?

Fat Facts

Fat is vital to human growth and development, particularly for the endurance athlete. As a double ironman triathlete, which takes approximately twenty-four hours to finish, Gary uses more fat than the average athlete does.

Athletes' bodies store about 50,000 to 60,000 calories of triglyceride energy; therefore, even the leanest have adequate fat storage to meet the metabolic demands of activity. However, the proportion of fat used for exercise is dependent on duration and intensity.

The importance of carbohydrates has already been discussed in chapters 1 and 3. Since the body can only slowly convert body fat stores into energy during exercise, maintaining high levels of muscle glycogen is essential for high-intensity exercise. Therefore, when muscle and liver levels are low, exercise intensity must be reduced to support the body's limited ability to convert fat into energy. In endurance-trained athletes like Gary and Jonathan, fat use is enhanced while carbohydrates are "spared," allowing them to exercise longer before becoming exhausted from glycogen depletion.

Fat is a great long-term energy source for distance events, providing 2,000–3,000 calories versus 1,500 calories of carbohydrate stored in muscle. It is also easier and lighter to carry around than carbohydrates, since carbohydrates store three times as much water weight. However, muscle fat works at only one-third the rate of carbohydrates for intense energy needs. Therefore, during strenuous training or competition, fats supplement carbohydrates only to supply ATP to the working muscle during high-intensity exercise.

The Vegetarian and Dietary Fats

Although some types of dietary fat have been linked to cardiovascular disease, obesity, hypertension, cancer, and possibly gall bladder disease, vegetarian diets are generally low in fat, saturated fat, and cholesterol and offer protection against these diseases. Vegetarian diets also tend to be higher in antioxidants such as vitamin C and E, carotenoids, phytochemicals, and fiber as well as have a higher concentration of folate, which reduces homocysteine levels, all of which have been shown to protect against disease.

Total serum cholesterol and low-density lipoprotein (LDL) cholesterol levels are usually lower in vegetarians, but high-density lipoproteins and triglyceride levels may vary depending on the type of vegetarian diet followed. In fact, some lacto-ovo, pesco-, and semi-vegetarians can get an excessive amount of fat and saturated fat, depending on the type and preparation of animal products selected.

Dietary Fats

Dietary fats come from three major groups: triglycerides, 95% of the fats we eat; phospholipids, which are soluble in fat and water and act as an emulsifier, like lecithin, which helps mix fat and water together by breaking fat globules into smaller ones; and sterols, the cholesterol and sex hormone fats, which assist in normal development and gender-related functioning.

Fats are essential for

▶ long-term energy use

▶ provision of the essential fatty acids, linoleic and linolenic

▶ transportation of the fat-soluble vitamins A, E, D, and K

▶ creating the flavors and palatable qualities of food to the palate

▶ aiding in satiety

Fats are a concentrated energy source, providing twice as many calories as protein or carbohydrates. Since the body is capable of manufacturing stored fat from extra dietary protein and carbohydrates, excessive fat intakes are unnecessary. In fact, an individual only needs about 3 to 6 grams (27–54 calories) of fat per day to accomplish fat's basic functions. The remainder fuels the athlete or is stored as adipose for "later use" in the less active person. Excess fat intake has been associated with the incidence of heart disease.

There are two major dietary fat groups: unsaturated and saturated fats. The saturated fats are solid at room temperature. These fats have been shown to increase total and low-density lipoprotein blood cholesterol levels. Some saturated fats are more hypercholesterolemic than others are. Stearic acid, a saturated fat found in meats and chocolate, does not appear to demonstrate this effect.

The unsaturated fats include polyunsaturated (PUFA) and mono-unsaturated fats. These fats have been shown to reduce total and LDL blood cholesterol levels. The major categories of PUFA include the Omega-6s from vegetable oils and the Omega-3s from fish oils. Large doses of the Omega-3s have been shown to lower plasma triglycerides but do not consistently lower total cholesterol levels. And if the diet contains more than 10% PUFA from the essential unsaturated fatty acid Omega-6, it can also lower the "good" cholesterol, high-density lipoprotein (HDL), which helps to "clean out" excess cholesterol in the body.

The World Health Organization (WHO), the American Heart Association, and other health organizations suggest limiting dietary fat to less than 30% of total calories and saturated fat to 10% of total calories. This means that an athlete following a 2,000-calorie program would limit fat intake to 600 calories (66 grams), of which 60 calories (6.6 grams) would come from saturated fat.

All foods contain a combination of fats. A chart with foods representing each group is on page 89.

Cholesterol

Cholesterol serves as the raw material for making bile. It is an important sterol fat in the structure of brain and nerve cells. Like lecithin, the body makes cholesterol, so it is not considered essential. It is found in animal products and foods prepared with animal products. Since elevated levels of cholesterol are a risk factor for heart disease and strokes, the American Heart Association recommends a dietary intake of 300 mg daily or less. This is not usually a concern to vegetarian athletes who limit or abstain from animal products.

▶ Sources of Saturated and Unsaturated Fats ◀

SATURATED FATS	MONOUNSATURATED FATS	POLYUNSATURATED FATS	HYDROGENATED FATS
Palm oil	Olive oil	Safflower oil	Cookies
Animal fats	Canola oil	Soybean oil	Crackers
Coconuts and coconut oil	Sunflower oil	Corn oil	Chips
Palm kernel oil	Peanuts and peanut oil	Sunflower oil	Fast foods
Cream	Avocados	Fish and fish oil	
Whole milk	Cashews	Almonds	
Shortening	Poultry	Cottonseed oil	
Stick margarine		Pecans	
Lard		Walnuts	
Cocoa butter		Liquid/soft margarine	
Hydrogenated oils		Mayonnaise	
Cheese		Sesame oil	

Essential Fats

The body uses carbohydrates, fat, or protein to make nearly all the fat it needs. Two polyunsaturated fatty acids essential to health that must be supplied by the diet are linoleic acid (Omega-6) from vegetable oils, seeds, nuts, and whole grains, and linolenic acid (Omega-3) from fatty fish, full-fat soy products, canola oil, and flaxseed. The body uses these fats to make hormone-like substances that control blood pressure and blood clot formation and regulate blood lipids and the substances that respond to infection and injury. They also serve as structural parts of cells. A deficiency can lead to growth problems, skin abnormalities, and kidney and liver disorders.

Diets that do not contain fish or eggs lack the two Omega-3s docosahexanoic acid (DHA) and EPA. Vegetarians may have lower blood levels, although not all studies confirm this. The essential fatty acid linolenic acid can be converted to DHA, although the conversion rates appear to be inefficient. High linoleic acid intakes interfere with the conversion. Diets too high in fat, especially from vegetable oils and processed foods, can inhibit the conversion of linolenic acid to DHA. Diets too low in fat may not provide enough. There are no Recommended Dietary Allowances for Omega-6s and Omega-3s, but scientists may agree to include them in the future. Ideally, the ratio between Omega-6 fatty acids and Omega-3s should be limited to 10:1 and preferably closer to 5:1. Vegetarians need to include good sources of linolenic acid in their diet.

▶ Sources of Linolenic Acid ◀

Flaxseed, 2 tbs	4.3 grams
Walnuts, 1 oz	1.9 grams
Soybeans, $\frac{1}{2}$ cup cooked	0.5 grams
Tofu, $\frac{1}{2}$ cup	0.4 grams
Walnut oil, 1 tbs	1.5 grams
Canola oil, 1 tbs	1.6 grams
Linseed oil, 1 tbs	7.6 grams
Soybean oil, 1 tbs	0.9 grams

Source: American Dietetic Association Position Statement, 1997.

Some great recipes including sources of the essential fatty acids are Charlene's Triple Axel Veggie Surprise (see below) and Erika's Trail Mix Snack, prepared with walnuts, soy nuts, and raisins.

Charlene's Triple Axel Veggie Surprise

Makes 2 servings

———

1 green onion

1 tbs fresh ginger

$\frac{1}{4}$ cup each frozen corn, peas, carrots (diced)

$\frac{1}{2}$ tin soybeans or adzuki beans

3 oz firm tofu*

1 tsp safflower oil

$\frac{1}{2}$–$\frac{3}{4}$ cup short-grain brown rice

1 tsp shoyu (or tamari sauce)

———

Sauté onion and ginger in safflower oil until onions are clear.
Add the veggies, beans, and tofu and mix for 2 minutes.
Finish by adding rice for 1–2 minutes. Stir in shoyu. Voilá!

▶ Nutrients per serving: 332 calories, 22 grams protein, 34
  grams carbohydrates, 15 grams fat, 2 grams saturated fat,
  3 grams monounsaturated fat, 7 grams linoleic fat, 3 grams
  sugar, 2 grams fiber

▶ Dietary composition: 24% protein, 38% carbohydrates,
  37% fat

▶ VSNG food servings: 1 veggie, 2 grains, 2 protein, $1\frac{1}{2}$ fats

▶ Good source of vitamin A, magnesium, iron, manganese;
  moderate source of vitamin B_1, folate, potassium, calcium,
  copper, selenium

*Food fitness note: Mori-Nu makes a low-fat tofu.

To Hydrogenate or Not...
That Is the Question

In an effort to reduce serum cholesterol levels, individuals have been
eliminating animal sources of fats, which contain primarily saturated
fat and cholesterol. In order for food manufacturers to replace the
saturated fat source with a palatable replacement, they have taken
unsaturated fats and saturated them by adding hydrogen to the
bonds on the fat molecule where they are missing, hence the process
known as hydrogenation.

A continuing source of conflict among scientific experts is the
result of the process of hydrogenation of unsaturated fats. Research
is still unsettled regarding the risk of saturating them to make them
behave like saturated fats in foods. Some research shows that during
the hydrogenation process, the normal stored form of fats in the body
is distorted to another chemical form called trans-fatty acids. These fats
may increase the risk of heart disease and cancer. The jury is still out.
My suggestion is to look for naturally low-saturated-fat products or to
consume nonhydrogenated products. Some of those foods are listed
in chapter 9. However, foods not listed in *The Vegetarian Sports*

Nutrition Guide food lists are sometimes not called "hydrogenated" on their labels. Therefore, hold back on that extra doughnut, Danish, french fries, and corn chips the next time you feel the urge to splurge!

How Do Athletes Size Up?

According to the latest national health surveys, the average American consumes about 36 to 37% total calories from fat: 13% saturated fat and 14% monounsaturated fat. The Diet and Health Committee of the National Academy of Sciences (the RDA people) recommends daily intakes of

▶ less than 30% total dietary fat

▶ less than 10% saturated fat

▶ less than 7% polyunsaturated fat (from nonhydrogenated sources)

▶ less than 13% monounsaturated fat

Previous studies showed that athletes from a variety of sports reported intakes of approximately 32 to 41% total calories from fat. The VSNG athletes appear to maintain a range of 6 to 28% total dietary fat in their daily diets.

Exercising Fat's Options

The value of fat for exercise is its storage capacity, about fifty times the amount of carbohydrate. Its primary role is to protect the body against depleting the body's 2,000-calorie carbohydrate stores in the form of muscle glycogen. The liver stores an additional 400 calories of glycogen, but that is mainly used to maintain blood glucose and fuel nervous system tissue.

Fats can never provide the total energy need without the help of carbohydrates. Although the supply of fats is almost unlimited, the ability of muscle to use it for energy is not. Fat utilization is apparently tied to the drop in blood glucose that occurs over time with exercise. Low carbohydrate stores will trigger greater fat utilization, so in endurance athletes this is a daily occurrence. It takes up to 45 hours to completely refuel carbohydrate reserves, and even longer when dietary carbohydrate intake is inadequate.

Typically, it's not fat itself that's the limiting factor in performance at low intensity, but it is related to the conditions that are necessary for the metabolism of fat, such as low blood sugar and glycogen. Consuming a high-fat diet may result in a larger proportion of fats used during exercise, but this diet limits the amount of carbohydrates stored, which are necessary for the complete oxidation of fats.

The degree to which fats are used is dependent on

▶ exercise intensity and duration

▶ diet

▶ endurance training history

▶ altered metabolic state

▶ possibly the use of caffeine and other ergogenic aids (see chapter 6)

Triglycerides are the body's primary stored form of fat. Triglycerides can be stored around the body's cells or within muscle cells. The ones stored in muscles are immediately available to fuel exercise. Adipose fat must be transported to the working muscle.

Of the three potential body fat sources, adipose, blood triglycerides, and free fatty acids, stored adipose and muscular fats are the only practical sources during exercise. Free fatty acids and blood triglycerides provide only a total of .75 grams (under 7 calories) and 8 grams (72 calories), respectively.

A process called lipolysis breaks down the fat molecule, transporting fatty acids away from adipose fat to be used by muscle. Intramuscular fat has been shown to decrease by 30 to 50% during 30km and 100km races. Because training can increase the capacity of the muscle to use fat, Gary, running a pace that is 70% VO2max for one hour, can derive up to 75% of his total energy requirement through fat.

Exercise levels of less than 50% VO2max mainly use slow-twitch muscle fibers and rely on the availability of free fatty acids for fuel. As exercise intensity increases, carbohydrates are used preferentially as a fuel source. Fast-twitch muscles prefer to use carbohydrates for energy; hence, the rate at which fat is used declines with exercise intensity. Training increases the fat-usage rate of fast-twitchers by changing their energy potential.

Training to Enhance Fat Metabolism

Endurance training affects the number of mitochondria (aerobic powerhouses) per cell and increases the amount of fat-burning enzymes. This training enables endurance athletes like Dave Scott, Ben Mathews, Gary Gromet, and Bob Abate to burn fat as an energy substrate and

▶ use oxygen more efficiently and exercise at a higher intensity with less respiratory effort

▶ use more oxygen at a given workload

▶ decrease the rate of glycogen use via "glycogen sparing"

▶ lower lactate production

That's why they can afford to eat higher-fat recipes like Heath's Skating Mexican Fiesta Meal (page 95) without any adverse effects. In fact, several of the VSNG athletes report enjoying Mexican-based tortilla, refried bean, and cheese combos after training. Some ways that fat-conscious individuals can save fat calories is to purchase fat-free refried beans, fat-free soy cheese, and low-fat tortillas (see the VSNG Foundation Food Lists).

Very little is known about the best ways to train to improve fat use. Two ways that may work are to thoroughly warm up prior to competition and to exercise in the cold. Beyond that, one can only speculate. Some other suggestions are to:

▶ Limit carbohydrate stores, stimulating the release of glucagon. Back-to-back "brick" workouts of run/swim, bike/run, or sport-specific training, and a workout immediately after at the gym, can also accomplish that goal.

▶ Use water as a fluid replacement in training. Limiting carbohydrate intake during training will encourage rapid adaptations to the fat system. Save the sport fluids for race time.

My favorite fat-pushing workouts are long, 90-minute-plus aerobic sessions of run/swim/run, run/bike/run/swim, or run/bike/gym. At a minimum, I end my longer runs with a few sets of squats with a weight bar, biceps with ten-pound dumbbells, and a lower, upper, and oblique (side) ab workout. I may also add a more comprehensive weight-training session on mid-distance 6- to 10-mile runs.

Heath's Skating Mexican Fiesta Meal

Makes 1 serving

———

1 flour tortilla*
½ can refried beans (Rosarita is Craig's favorite brand)*
1 small can of corn
2 handfuls of lettuce
2 tsp Newman's olive oil (Craig's favorite brand)
salsa (mild is Craig's favorite)

———

Warm tortilla in microwave. Mix and heat beans and corn in 2 tsp olive oil. Spread on tortilla. Top with lettuce and salsa. When Craig has rice, he adds that to the bean/corn mixture, too!

▶ Nutrients per serving: 485 calories, 19 grams protein, 63 grams carbohydrates, 19 grams fat, 3 grams saturated fat, 5 grams monounsaturated fat, 7 grams linoleic fat, 9 grams fiber

▶ Dietary composition: 15% protein, 50% carbohydrates, 35% fat

▶ VSNG food servings: ¼ vegetable, 4 grains, 3 fats

▶ Good source of vitamin K, folate, iron; moderate source of vitamin B_1, potassium, phosphorus, magnesium, manganese

*Food fitness note: whole wheat organic tortillas; Shari's makes fat-free refried beans

A Load of Fat

Recently, several studies have stirred some controversy by suggesting that athletes may perform better on high-fat diets, 30% fat or higher. This "fat-loading" research includes one 1983 cycling study and two impressive 1994 running and cycling studies, which demonstrated that high-fat diets of 85%, 38% and 70% fat respectively contradicted previous work regarding the necessity of high-carbohydrate diets for peak performance. Unfortunately, despite increasing time until exhaustion, increasing VO2max, and improving performance times, these studies had several flaws, including lack of randomization and other inconsistencies.

"The drawbacks of high-fat diets outweigh any potential benefits," according to a *Sports Medicine Digest* article by Ellen Coleman, sports nutrition expert and author of *Eating for Endurance*. These drawbacks include

▶ the risk of sudden death and heart rhythm disturbances due to protein losses from the heart and potassium depletion

▶ increased blood cholesterol levels, which may increase the athlete's risk for heart disease

▶ difficulty in digesting high-fat diets

▶ two weeks or more needed to adapt to high-fat diets

▶ impaired ability to perform at high intensity

In fact, any programs that exceed the recommended 30% total caloric fat intake appear to increase other risk factors for heart disease, stroke, and other diseases.

Despite the limitations, this research may indicate that some athletes—highly trained ones—may benefit from additional fat. Some athletes consistently limit their amount of dietary fat intake to extremes for a variety of reasons. Perhaps some athletes have trouble meeting their calorie needs on their normal high-carb diets. Others consume low-nutrient-density, high-carbohydrate diets, and hence find that they don't feel as fit on high carbs. With the additional fat and/or fat density of the new diet, it allows them to meet their needs and improve performance.

Medium-Chain Triglycerides

Since increasing fatty acids during exercise will spare muscle glycogen, ways to increase them through supplements or increased fat intake without compromising carbohydrate intake can be beneficial to endurance performance. Medium-chain triglycerides (MCTs) may fit that bill.

Unlike other fats, MCTs do not delay gastric emptying or absorption. They are broken down in the stomach, metabolized as quickly as glucose, and may even supply an alternative energy source for muscle during endurance exercise. They occur naturally only in milk fat, where only a small fraction is found. MCTs are made synthetically by hydrolysis of coconut oil followed by other chemical means. They have a low melting point and are liquid at room temperature. MCTs have eight calories per gram, compared to fat at nine calories per gram.

Since they are smaller and more soluble than long-chain triglycerides, MCTs require less bile and pancreatic juices for digestion and absorption. Also, they are not incorporated into the fat transportation vehicles called chylomicrons like other fats. After they leave the intestines, they enter the liver faster with the protein vehicle albumin. Unlike other fats, their use in the mitochondria is not dependent on carnitine. And although MCTs are a saturated fat, they appear to reduce cholesterol.

Recently, MCTs have been shown to be beneficial to athletes. One study showed the benefits at high intensities through infusion techniques. Infused MCTs bypass the liver, allowing the skeletal muscle to use the available substrate and spare muscle glycogen. Ingesting MCTs by mouth may not fuel the exercising muscle. Another recent study showed faster time trials when compared to individuals who consumed only carbohydrate products. Thirty grams appears to be the dose used in these studies. Even though MCTs are used more rapidly, especially when consumed with carbohydrates (as in liquid form), most individuals cannot consume more than 30 grams without suffering from GI discomfort and diarrhea.

Alternative Fats

In an effort to reduce dietary fats but maintain the textural properties of fat, the development of alternative ingredients and food-processing methods has produced substitutions to reduce or eliminate all fats in food products. According to an analysis by Kraft General Foods, by using alternative fats, total fat calorie intake can be reduced from 36 to 30% (10 grams per day) to meet health recommendations. The NutraSweet Company reported the impact from the use of Simplesse, a protein-based fat replacement that can reduce the daily saturated fat and cholesterol content by 21% and 9% respectively, and increase the protein content from 16 to 17%.

Many of the fat replacements in use today are a result of heating, acidifying, and blending common food ingredients such as carbohydrates, milk and egg proteins, and/or water to replicate the textural properties of fat. Since many use standard ingredients and processing methods, they do not normally require approval by the Food and Drug Administration (FDA). Other products feature fat reduction technologies or new ingredients, which may require FDA approval. Examples of some everyday foods that include alternative fats are fat-free salad dressings, baked goods, chips, cheeses, and frozen desserts and yogurt.

Some of the names and uses for fat replacements can be found in the Fat Replacement Chart on page 99.

Food Fats

Fats are a natural component of most foods, to varying degrees. They are often added in processing to make foods taste and smell good to the consumer. Fatty foods have a major role in inhibiting gastric emptying, therefore leaving you feeling satiated or satisfied after mealtime. That is why fatty foods are not recommended prior to competition. They stay in the system too long and can cause GI distress, nausea, and fatigue.

In light of all the research on fat and performance, some fat in food and athletes' diets is essential for good health. Many of the recipes throughout the book provide a healthy proportion of fats. Several VSNG favorite snack choices also contain fat, but from the desirable less saturated type. Many of the athletes rely on these foods to provide essential fats in their diets when compared with others who add unnecessary fats to foods, such as sauces, oils, and greases, with high-fat cooking methods.

One benefit to having more fat in meals and snack foods is preventing overconsumption. That's why professional and Olympic figure skater Charlene Wong Williams prefers to eat regular popcorn and chips instead of the low-fat variety. Some of the highest-fat meals in this book are a favorite by Dina Head called Head's Slam Dunk Fish Dish (see page 102) and Brown's Curling Kenyan Tortilla (page 103), both found at the end of this chapter.

► Fat Replacement Chart ◄

Type	Composition	Calories/Gram	Trade Names
Carbohydrate-based	Dextrin, modified food starches, polydextrose and gums. Heat-stable and can be used in cooking; does not melt.	1–4	Maltrin, STA-SLIM 143, Polydextrose, Avicel
Protein-based	Milk and/or egg white proteins, water, sugar, pectin, and citric acid. Cannot be used in frying but can be used in baked goods, lasagna, pizza and cheesecake, mayonnaise, sour cream, salad dressings, desserts, yogurt, and cheese.	1–2	Simplesse
Fat-based	Monoglycerides, diglyceride emulsifiers, modified food starch and guar gum in a milk base. Used in cakes and cookies.	5.1	N-Flate
	Vegetable oils, used in smaller quantities to reduce fat; cake mixes, cookies, icings, and vegetable dairy products.	9	Dur-Lo
	Reduced-calorie triglyceride. Used in candy and confectionery coatings.	5	Caprenin
	Formed by esterification of sucrose with fatty acids from oil. Resembles fat in frying, cooking, and baking. Since it is not absorbed in the digestive tract, fat-soluble vitamin absorption may be inhibited. Vitamins A, D, E, and K are added to foods with Olestra (i.e., chips); may also cause cramping and diarrhea in some individuals.	0	Olestra

Note: Other fat replacements are under development but have not been submitted to the FDA for review.

Spotlight Athlete

Gary Gromet
Double ironman triathlete

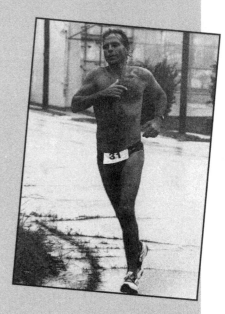

Age: 53

12 years pesco-vegetarian

Reason for becoming vegetarian:
"Healthier diet."

Advantages of being vegetarian:
"Since I am healthier, I am
able to participate in my
sports at an optimal level."

Challenges to being vegetarian:
none

Alcohol: four glasses of wine or
beer per week

Medications: none

Supplements: vitamins E and C, magnesium, alphalipoic acid,
glucosamine, glutamine, ferrochal bisglycinate, lycopene,
phytoflavonoids, CoQ10, creatine, carnitine, melatonin,
grapeseed, ginseng, ginkgo biloba, tribulus tennestris, whey
protein powder, Cytomax sport drink

Favorite prerace meal: Parillo Bar

Favorite snacks: German bread, sweet potatoes, Parillo Bars,
frozen protein shakes, roasted soybeans

Favorite one-pot meal: grilled tofu cheese on whole wheat
German bread

Spotlight Athlete

Jonathan Didonato
*Guinness Book record holder
for long-distance butterfly swimming*

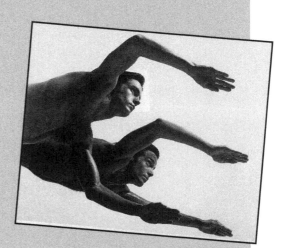

Age: 44

18 years
   semivegetarian

*Reason for becoming
   vegetarian:*
"Stamina and
to excel in sports."

*Challenges to being
   vegetarian:* none

Alcohol: none

Supplements: spirulina and bee pollen

Favorite prerace meal: barley

Favorite snacks: chocolate and power shakes

Favorite one-pot meal: Didonato's Swimming Rice Primavera
   (page 104)

Head's Slam Dunk Fish Dish

Makes 4 servings

$^{1}/_{2}$ tsp garlic powder
$^{1}/_{2}$ tsp salt
$^{1}/_{2}$ tsp black pepper
$^{1}/_{2}$ tsp red pepper
$^{1}/_{2}$ tsp basil
$^{1}/_{2}$ pound shrimp, shelled and deveined
$^{1}/_{4}$ stick margarine
1 16 oz package frozen broccoli spears
$^{1}/_{2}$ cup water
2 tsp margarine
$^{1}/_{2}$ tsp salt

For shrimp dish:

Mix seasonings with shrimp prior to cooking. Sauté shrimp in margarine. Drain shrimp after cooking.

For broccoli dish:

Steam broccoli for 10–15 minutes. Mix broccoli and shrimp together. Bon appetit!

▶ Nutrients per serving: 361 calories, 27 grams protein, 8 grams carbohydrates, 25 grams fat, 5 grams saturated fat, 10 grams monounsaturated fat, 7 grams linoleic fat, 2 grams sugar, 4 grams fiber

▶ Dietary composition: 30% protein, 9% carbohydrates, 62% fat*

▶ VSNG food servings: 1 vegetable, 3.5 protein, 5 fats

▶ Good source of vitamin B_{12}, C, K, folate, chloride; moderate source of vitamin A, B_3, D, E, sodium, potassium, phosphorus, magnesium, and iron

*Food fitness note: Perhaps the fat helps Dina satisfy her tummy after a hard game or practice. You can reduce the fat by eliminating most of the margarine. You can also use an unhydrogenated soy margarine to eliminate hydrogenated fats and increase isoflavones (phytochemicals—see chapter 7) for health.

Brown's Curling Kenyan Tortilla

*Makes 1 serving (Have an extra tortilla ready
for sharing any leftovers with a friend!)*

1 onion, diced

1 tomato, diced

1 red and 1 green pepper, diced

$\frac{1}{2}$ cup tomato paste

1 cup kidney beans

3 cloves garlic, minced

Tabasco sauce (optional)

cayenne pepper

1 tortilla

2 tsp corn oil

In a large frying pan, sauté onions, tomatoes, and peppers in corn oil. Add kidney beans and tomato paste. Add garlic, Tabasco sauce, and cayenne pepper. "Put the concoction into a tortilla and eat up!"

▶ Nutrients per serving: 570 calories, 24 grams protein, 96 grams carbohydrates, 13 grams fat, 1 gram saturated fat, 2 grams monounsaturated fat, 6 grams linoleic acid, 7 grams sugar, 21 grams fiber

▶ Dietary composition: 16% protein, 64% carbohydrates, 20% fat

▶ VSNG food servings: $3\frac{1}{2}$ vegetables, 4 grains, $2\frac{1}{2}$ fats

▶ Good source of vitamin A, C, B_6, B_3, folate, potassium, phosphorus, iron, copper; moderate source of vitamin B_1, B_2, pantothenic acid, sodium, calcium, magnesium, zinc, manganese, selenium

▼

Didonato's Swimming Rice Primavera
Makes 2 servings

1 cup broccoli

1 cup corn

1 cup peas

1 cup lima beans

1 red pepper, diced

1 cup watercress

2 cups long-grain brown rice, cooked

2 tsp olive oil

———

Sauté vegetables in olive oil al dente. Mix with rice. Voilá!

▶ Nutrients per serving: 493 calories, 17 grams protein, 95 grams carbohydrates, 7 grams fat, 12 grams fiber

▶ Dietary composition: 14% protein, 74% carbohydrates, 12% fat

▶ VSNG food servings: 1 vegetable, 6 grains, 1 fat

▶ Good source of vitamin A, C, B_1, B_6, K, folate, pantothenic acid, biotin, potassium, phosphorus, magnesium, iron, manganese, copper

6

Thirst Quenchers

BEN RICHARDSON, a world-class Laser sailor and four-year vegetarian, was vegan for a year and a half until a ten-day trip abroad without protein forced him to turn to chicken and fish. Previously heavy, Ben, at 22 and a Harvard grad, became a vegetarian to help him reach his ideal competitive weight. He remains a semivegetarian for the same reason.

Other than an occasional beer, Ben only "cheats" on his healthy program with ice cream for snacks. For his high-power anaerobic sport, Ben supplements with chromium and creatine. His typical day includes his favorite prerace meal of oatmeal, soy milk, and soy protein; salad and protein-rich vegetables for lunch; a Balance Bar for an afternoon snack; and fish for dinner. His favorite Mexican-style meal resembles Craig Heath's favorite one-pot meal in chapter 5 on page 95.

Another athlete who manages her best competitive weight with a vegetarian diet is Charlene Wong Williams, an Olympic and professional skater who performs and competes on another state of water—sheets of ice. Charlene also became a vegetarian to feel better and healthier and improve her appearance and moods.

The sport of professional figure skating demands all the elements: beauty, talent, and athletic ability. For this, Charlene, a primarily vegan vegetarian, and her vegetarian "former-skating" husband, use no refined sugars or flours, artificial sweeteners, or caffeine in their plentiful and diverse "in variety and textures" diet.

With up to 4 hours of ice training and 2½ hours of aerobic conditioning daily, Charlene supports her energy needs with a day beginning with hot cereals, whole grains, nut butters, and rice milk. Afternoon meals often include greens, tempeh, stir-fry and tofu, vegetable juice, fruit or chips, and steamed veggies. She never drinks alcohol and takes no supplements. The only challenge she sees is the commitment to planning meals, especially while traveling.

These "water-based" athletes can really appreciate the value of fluids in their sports. During the typical Laser time trial, Ben's strapped in a cockpit, knees hanging off the boat's side, for a 1- or 2½-hour race, three times a day, sometimes for 8 to 9 days in the hot sun. How does he get enough fluid while competing? He says, "Very carefully!" He also prepares by consuming about 32 ounces prior to competition time.

You can lead a horse to water, but you can't make him drink . . .

Fluids are as important as food when it comes to sport. Water is vital for all lives every day in every way. We can last several months without some vitamins and minerals, about 8 weeks without food, but only a few days without water. Just ask Ben, Jane, Gary, and other endurance athletes. Bob Abate, the deca-ironman, can testify to how valuable water and other fluids are during his 12-day race. The truth is, water is critical for all athletes at all times.

About 60% of the adult body is composed of the liquid essential, H_2O. Even the "dry" portions like bone, muscle, and teeth are 20%, 75%, and 10% water, respectively. About two-thirds of the water is found inside the cells as intracellular fluid. The rest is outside the cells, primarily in blood, as extracellular fluid. Fluid found outside but between cells is called interstitial fluid. The body manages how much water is in these compartments by maintaining control over nutrients and minerals found inside and outside the cell.

How does water help us function? Water

▶ transports nutrients in blood

▶ provides a medium and assists with chemical reactions in cells and carries away the waste products formed during those reactions

▶ acts as a shock absorber in joints and around the spinal cord

- lubricates the digestive tract and tissues moistened with mucus
- surrounds and cushions an unborn child
- regulates body temperature (when sweat evaporates, heat is released, leaving the body cooler)
- acts as a solvent to form solutions (Like a preacher, water "marries" positively charged substances to negatively charged substances. Sodium chloride—table salt—is an example of this. Other substances can also "divorce" or "dissociate" in the presence of water. One example is electrolytes.)

Fluid Needs of Athletes

Normal adult water requirements are estimated at one milliliter per calorie of energy, or about 9 to 12 cups per day. Most of the water we need comes through a variety of beverages and food. Fruits and vegetables contain 85 to 95% water. Chef Hanners' Tempeh Gumbo is an example of a dish with about two cups of fluid per serving (see page 108).

During exercise, as little as 1% body weight loss of water can cause discomfort, thirst, and loss of appetite. A 4% loss in body weight causes lethargy, anxiety, nausea, and irritability. At 8%, dizziness, cyanosis, indistinct speech, weakness, and mental confusion set the stage for eventual heat exhaustion, heatstroke, and death if not treated. Endurance athletes training or competing in warm, humid conditions are particularly at risk for heat-related stress.

Water Loss

The major source of water loss from the body is the urine, followed by feces and evaporation from the lungs and skin. Typical urine output is 1 to 2 liters per day. The waste products found in urine are urea and other nitrogen-containing products from protein breakdown, ketones from fat breakdown, phosphates, sulfates, and other electrolytes. When protein exceeds requirements, the excess is broken down and nitrogen must be excreted in the urine. More than 95% of water is reabsorbed before the feces are eliminated.

Water losses due to sweat and lungs vary considerably. For the inactive person in a cool environment, losses do not exceed 1 ½ liters per day. In a dry environment in an airplane or desert, losses can be 2 cups per hour. With heavy training in a hot environment, it could increase tenfold.

Hanners' Tempeh Gumbo

Makes 4 servings

1 onion, diced

2 stalks celery, diced

1 red and 1 green pepper, diced

2 carrots, diced

½ cup okra

2 cups tomatoes

1 cup rice

1 quart vegetable stock

1 package tempeh, chopped

1 tsp cayenne

1 tsp Old Bay seasoning

1 tbs gumbo filé powder

1 tbs olive oil

In a large stockpot, sauté all vegetables in olive oil until tender. Add tomatoes and stew, covered, for 2 minutes. Add rice and stock. Reduce to a simmer. Add chopped tempeh and seasonings. Cook 25 minutes.

▶ Nutrients per serving: 340 calories, 13 grams protein, 55 grams carbohydrates, 8 grams fat, 3 grams monounsaturated fat, 2.5 grams linoleic fat, 6 grams sugar, 6 grams fiber

▶ Good source of vitamin A, C, manganese; moderate source of vitamin K, folate, potassium, magnesium

▶ Dietary composition: 15% protein, 63% carbohydrates, 22% fat

▶ VSNG food servings: 1.25 vegetable, 3 grains, 1 fat

The American College of Sports Medicine (ACSM) position contains specific points regarding fluid guidelines. Some of these have been included in the Guidelines for Fluid Replacement.

▶ Guidelines for Fluid Replacement ◀

TIME	TYPE	AMOUNT	COMMENTS
24 hours before training and competition	Cool mineral water and/or sport drinks*, frozen fruit pops	To maintain hydration	Limit alcohol, caffeinated drinks, and excess dietary fiber
2 hours before training and competition	Cool water*	16–20 oz	Sport drinks that are 4–8% (14 grams per 8 oz) carbohydrates; 1 gm/kg body weight glycerol in 1.5 liters fluid
10–15 minutes before training and competition	Cool water*	Up to 2 cups	As tolerated (test your system during training)
Every 10–15 minutes during exercise	Cool water and/or sport drink*	4–6 oz, 25–30 grams carbs every ½ hour; .5-.7 grams sodium/liter water for 1 hour+ events	Sport drink with electrolytes for hot weather, up to 1 gram sodium/hour for ultraendurance athletes
Immediately after exercise	Water and/or sweet fluids*	2 cups for each pound lost (up to 150% of total fluids lost)	Limit caffeine, alcohol, plain water, or sweet fortified drinks; drink until you are regularly urinating and the urine is clear (however, vitamin supplements will make the color darker)

*Drinks should be 59–72° F and flavored to promote fluid replacement.

Fluid Ergogenics

Staying hydrated makes you perform better regardless of your sport. Impairments can be prevented by consuming fluids before, during, and after the training session, but are not limited to these factors. Fluids also need to be sensitive to taste, gastric emptying, and absorption and should consider the addition of glucose, sodium, and amino acids to enhance absorption.

Electrolytes

Electrolytes are popular additions to sport drinks like Gatorade. Electrolytes are minerals such as sodium, chloride, and potassium that regulate the distribution of fluid in body compartments and are important in nerve conduction, which leads to muscle contraction. Hyperhydration, dehydration, excessive consumption of sodium, and kidney problems cause flaws in electrolyte regulation.

Deficiencies in potassium, chloride, or sodium can cause serious medical problems such as hypertension, hyponatremia (low blood sodium), poor appetite, muscle cramps, confusion, apathy, constipation, and even irregular heartbeat. Athletes with eating disorders or stomach flu, low-calorie eaters, athletes who perspire excessively, and hypertensives on certain medications are at risk for electrolyte disturbances. Imbalances also occur during the initial stage of acclimation to heat, during prolonged, repeated exposure to training in hot, humid climates, and during long-distance events. Hyponatremia has been observed in long-distance triathlons, ultramarathons, and even tennis. Up to 1 gram of sodium per hour may be indicated for some ultraendurance athletes who are at risk.

Although no RDA has been established for sodium and potassium, daily dietary recommendations can be found in chapter 7. Sport drinks add approximately 50 to 110 mg of sodium per 8-ounce serving. Potassium is added in amounts of 25–45 milligrams. These needs can also be met through foods; however, in long-distance running or triathlon races, most foods are difficult to consume during the event.

Carbohydrates

The addition of carbohydrates to fluid replacement drinks is recommended for events lasting more than an hour, since plain water cannot restore energy needs. Water absorption causes plasma osmolality (particles per kilogram of solvent) to fall, suppresses thirst, and increases urine output. Data also suggest that 150% or more of weight loss in fluids may be required to achieve normal hydration within 6 hours following exercise.

Consuming at least 45 grams of carbohydrates each hour for events lasting more than an hour can improve performance. The maximal rate at which carbohydrates can be utilized is about 60 to 75 grams per hour, but differs from individual to individual. So if you're considering drinking and eating sport drinks, sport gels, and bars "on the run" at your next marathon, think again. Any distance runner will tell you about their worst marathon bathroom experience when they consumed too many sport drinks, sport gels, fluids, bars, and fruits while racing. The best time to consume these sugars is 25 to 30 grams every $\frac{1}{2}$ hour via a sport drink, sport gel, and beer if desired and tolerated.

The concentration of carbohydrates and variety of simple sugars in sport drinks varies. A combination of sucrose, glucose, fructose, and glucose polymers such as maltodextrin are included. Glucose polymers are chains of simple sugars linked together to provide more glucose without compromising gastric emptying. The addition of sugars can hinder or help performance. For some athletes, the presence of specific types of sugars, such as fructose, may cause cramping and diarrhea and hinder performance. Since sugar attracts water into the intestine, cramping, diarrhea, and dehydration are common side effects of getting too much.

In 1990, Fogoros coined the term "runner's trots" after a marathoner had described a bout of abdominal cramping and bloody diarrhea. The symptoms commonly associated with runner's diarrhea are lower abdominal cramping, an urge to defecate, and an increased frequency of bowel movements, rectal bleeding, and diarrhea. When runners lose more than 4% of their body weight during competition, they are much more likely to experience gastrointestinal symptoms.

Glucose in sport drinks has also been found to stimulate sodium and water absorption. Sodium is required for glucose transport, and chloride is preferred to maximize fluid absorption. Adding amino acids to a glucose-electrolyte drink may also enhance fluid absorption.

The density of carbohydrates also influences fluid absorption. The best concentration is 4 to 8% carbohydrates (14 grams per 8 oz). Since most sport drinks contain 6 to 7% carbohydrates (60–70 grams per liter), the consumption of one liter per hour will meet the athlete's needs. These fluids include most sport drinks. Beverages containing more than 7% carbohydrates are associated with slower absorption rates and increase the risk of GI distress. Soda and juice usually exceed this limit.

The Electrolytes

Sweat contains more sodium and chloride than other minerals. Although sweat electrolytes are substantially lower than blood values, athletes who train for more than 2 hours each day can lose considerable amounts of sodium chloride. The sodium content of sport drinks does not directly affect the rate of fluid absorption but can help to maintain the physiological drive for thirst, reduce the contribution of blood sodium required in the gut prior to absorption, and help to maintain plasma volume during exercise.

Amino Acids

Amino acids are added to drinks to stimulate sodium and water absorption and provide additional nutritional value. The effect of combining amino acids and sugars on water and salt absorption is additive. Drinks like Perform have added the amino acids glutamine, the branched chain amino acids, and A-acetyl cysteine to their formula.

Chemical Attraction

Water acts as a buffer to regulate pH. Chemical reactions in the body are very sensitive to changes in pH. Units of pH range from 1 to 14. Most reactions in the body occur at a pH of 7.4. If body fluids become too basic or too acidic, chemical reactions do not proceed efficiently.

A molecule that *releases* hydrogen in water is called an acid. A substance that *accepts* hydrogen is called a base. When the hydrogen content of a solution is low (pH high), the solution is alkaline or base. When acids or bases are added, buffers are the substances that resist changes in pH. Body water and dissolved electrolytes act as buffers to help regulate pH. Some athletes take supplements to buffer their pH when water changes, muscle exhaustion, lactic acid buildup (from the end product of anaerobic glycolysis), or nutritional deficiencies have affected their performance. Their effectiveness is discussed in chapter 8.

Other Fluids

Women, older individuals, and athletes are prone to urinary tract infections (UTIs). For decades, folk wisdom taught the public to drink cranberry-derived beverages to reduce bacterial infections of the bladder. As early as 1914, cranberry investigations indicated that cranberries, rich in benzoic acid, were secreted as hippuric acid in the urine. Studies from the 1920s through the 1970s suggested that acidification of the urine was the proposed mechanism by which cranberry juice produced a bacteriostatic effect, but recent studies show otherwise. Cranberry juice actually inhibits bacterial adherence to mucosal surfaces. Both cranberry and blueberry juices had this effect when compared to other fruit juices. A recent study showed that a dose of 300 ml of cranberry juice daily for four to eight weeks could make a difference.

Caffeine High

Caffeine has a long history of use in athletic competition. A "legal" drink until the 1970s, caffeine was shown to significantly improve cycling performance after consuming moderate doses. Following reports and articles written for popular magazines suggesting ten-minute Personal Records (PRs) for the 2:30 marathoner, the International Olympic Committee (IOC) banned the use of caffeine in international competition. The tolerance set by the IOC for caffeine concentration in the urine is 12 micrograms/ml. It's not easy to reach the 12 mcg/ml IOC limit. Even when a 70-kilogram athlete drinks four to six mugs of "drip" coffee an hour before a 1 1/2 hour training session, it will barely approach the limit. Caffeine doses below 9 mg/kg (630 mg caffeine for the 70-kg athlete) are well below the IOC limit.

Caffeine Theory 101

Since all body tissues soak up caffeine, it's difficult to isolate the effects of caffeine on muscle, fat, and the central nervous system (CNS). Different forms of exercise are affected by caffeine differently. Caffeine initially "pumps" our minds, dilates blood vessels, and helps the lungs to bring more oxygen to muscles. It speeds up the metabolism of sugars and fats from blood (instead of the muscles) and increases adrenaline, the "flight-fight" competitive response hormone that gets us ready for action.

Caffeine also has an ergogenic (energizing) effect on the

▶ liver, giving the athlete the initial blood "sugar pump" sensation

▶ skeletal muscle, getting calcium to be released to make the muscles work sooner and recover quicker from a contraction

▶ muscle fibers, assisting contraction, taking the pressure off the athlete, and reducing the perceived exertion (RPE) while exercising "under caffeine's influence"

▶ blood, by providing more fat and sparing muscle glycogen

Reports specific to the elite and recreational athlete have shown that a range of 3 to 13 mg/kg prior to endurance exercise has been shown to improve performance.

The downside to the cup of java is diarrhea and heart palpitations. Chronic caffeine consumption has been linked to the elevation of serum cholesterol, fibrocystic breast disease, and premenstrual syndrome (PMS). A list of beverages and foods containing caffeine is in the table on page 115.

> To calculate your potential ergogenic caffeine dose,
>> Take your body weight
>> Divide it by 2.2 to get kilograms of body weight
>> Multiply this by 3–6 mg
>> Find the drink and/or foods that meet this dose
>
> So if you weigh 150 pounds, you divide this by 2.2 and get approximately 70 kilograms body weight. 70 kilograms times 3 mg = 210 milligrams caffeine. Find the drink and/or food that meets your need and try it before a training session or two. A cup of coffee (150 mg), chocolate espresso Clif Bar (33 mg), and an iced tea (22–36 mg) would work. Don't wait until race day!

▶ Caffeine Content in Food, Beverages, and Medicines ◀

ITEM	MG/ SERVING
Coffee—5-oz cup	
Brewed	110–150
Instant	40–108
Decaf	2–5
Tea—5-oz cup	
Instant	12–28
Iced—12 oz	22–36
Cocoa	6
Soda—12 oz	
Mountain Dew	54
Coke or Diet Coke	46
Pepsi	38
Milk chocolate—1 oz	6
Sport Fuels	
Chocolate Espresso Clif Bar	33

ITEM	MG/ SERVING
Clif Shot, chocolate espresso	20
Pocket Rocket, chocolate	50
Power Gel, strawberry-banana	25
Balance Bar, mocha	15
PowerBar, chocolate	15
Gu gel	20
Stoker Bar, cocoa	5
No-Doz	100
Vivarin	200
Anacin	32
Excedrin	65
Midol	32
Triaminic	30
Dexatrim	200

Bottoms Up

Recent research suggests that a moderate daily alcohol intake may have a beneficial effect on health. However, alcohol abuse and dependence among nonathletes is as high as 24%. Athletes, too, have been known to indulge in alcohol consumption for a variety of reasons. These include reducing anxiety levels prior to competition, relaxing after training sessions, rejoicing after racing, or enjoying as a meal beverage.

Some sports, such as long-distance running, have been associated with problem drinking. In one recent study, running was shown to be a healthy substitution in a person prone to alcoholic behavior and may even aid in alcohol recovery. It's unclear if the chicken came before the egg . . . if running cut the drinking down or drinking induced less frequent exercise.

Some athletes feel that as long as they exercise, alcohol has no consequences. Actually, alcohol can be detrimental to athletic performance. Ten of the fifteen VSNG athletes reported drinking alcoholic beverages. Consumption ranged from seldom to a daily glass of wine or beer. So perhaps it is possible to enjoy a glass of "cheer" here and there and perform your best. Some of the best ways to work in a "cool one" are described in chapter 10.

Despite 7 calories from each gram of alcohol consumed, the muscles cannot use it as an energy source. In fact, while the body is processing alcohol, it limits the amount of sugar it releases to the bloodstream. This causes hypoglycemia (low blood sugar) and fatigue. Drinking alcohol may also contribute to hypothermia during cold weather. So for endurance athletes who think they can "carboload" (see chapter 4) on high-carbohydrate beer and wine, this is not the case.

Since dehydration can hurt the athlete's performance and alcohol causes dehydration, a night out on the town before a big race is not a great move! Alcohol, like caffeine, acts as a diuretic, causing increased urination and water loss. To metabolize 1 ounce of alcohol, the body requires 8 ounces water. In addition, energy-assisting B vitamins are required to process alcohol. Therefore, vegetarian athletes and other active-minded drinkers cannot afford to lose their valuable B's when healthy muscles are the first priority.

If you plan to spend a "night on the town," keep the following in mind:

▶ Drink 1 cup water for every alcoholic drink consumed to prevent the effects of dehydration. A drink is equal to a 12-ounce beer, 4 ounces of wine, or 1.5 ounces of 80 proof liquor.

▶ Get extra B's in the diet by consuming whole grains with bean dip, cereals with fortified soy milk, and whole-grain pretzels and snacks.

▶ Consume beer and wine instead of hard liquor. At least you'll get some carbs, chromium in beer, and iron in wine.

▶ Don't skip meals to consume a liquid diet.

▶ Don't choose to party the night before a big event. Consuming alcohol can lead to indigestion; nausea and vomiting; muscle, heart, brain, and esophagus abnormalities; and liver damage.

The "New Age" of Beverages

In 1997, *New Product News* reported 992 new ways to quench your thirst. Total U.S. consumption of beverages will reach close to 2 billion dollars in retail sales. Best-selling beverages are "traditional" soft drinks, bottled water, sport drinks, tea, and fruit beverages.

Drinking with a Purpose

America's obsession with health and fitness has encouraged a new league of drinks to splash onto the market. A public concern for tap water led to the bottled water craze, which doubles its market share, flavors, and ingredients yearly. Water joins another top-growing category, sport drinks, whose sales are expected to top $1 billion in 1999.

In addition to sugar and electrolytes, antioxidants, B vitamins, amino acids, and glycerol have also been added to some sport drinks like Perform and ProHydrator to give the athletes a performance edge. Despite the "New-Age" sport isotonics, Gatorade and now

Gatorade Frost continue to be the most popular brands. Wine has also become the year's new health drink, since its consumption has been shown to contribute to a healthy heart.

Several companies, including Hansen's, have also responded to this thirsty demand by providing a new variety of unusual blends and medicinal tonics. Even 100% fruit juices have been replaced with fruit and vegetable juice blends that contain caffeine or are fortified with vitamins, minerals, and fiber. One-stop liquid meals such as dairy-free Balanced are replacing food to meet the demands of an active lifestyle "on the run."

In addition to recreational fluids, sport drinks, and liquid food, a radical but legal group of fluids has emerged on the drinking scene.

Lifestyle Beverages

From nutrition basics 101 to a legal alternative to psychoactive drugs, the new drink lineup appears to be picking up where Snapple's exotic iced teas and other unusual recreational drinks left off. These beverages already have a $2 billion market. In Japan, one company, Aisho Pharmaceuticals, sells two million bottles of Lipovitan daily, a vitamin-fortified juice claiming to help counteract the effects of everything from excessive drinking and working to aging.

Beyond producing a caffeine high, these drinks often include "natural" vitamins and minerals, amino acids, herb extracts, and other ingredients that allegedly stimulate energy alertness or mind-altering effects. Unfortunately, many of these substances have not been subjected to adequate, controlled testing nor been proven to be effective or nontoxic. However, others may be safe and have a legitimate place in fitness, health, and disease prevention.

"Fringe beverages," designed to replace traditional mind-altering drugs and alcohol, are variants of sport and caffeinated energy beverages. The 3 G's, guarana, ginseng, and ginkgo biloba, as well as some mind-altering herbs such as St. John's wort and ma huang, supplement popular brands of soda, tea, juice, and fitness drinks. The purpose and safety of some of the herbs and additives can be found in the chart at the end of this chapter. Additional information on herbs can be found in chapter 8.

▲ Fluid and Lifestyle Beverages ▲

Type	Calories	Proteins	Carb*	Sugar	Fat	Fiber	Sugar Source	Extras
Sport Drinks								
Gatorade, 8 oz. Quaker Oats	50	0	14	14	0	0	Sucrose, glucose	Sodium, potassium, chloride, phosphorus
All Sport, 8 oz. Pepsi	70	0	19	19	0	0	High-fructose corn syrup	B vitamins B_1, B_3, B_6, B_{12}, folate, pantothenic acid
Powerade, 8 oz. Coca-Cola	70	0	19	19	0	0	High-fructose corn syrup, maltodextrin	Sodium, potassium
Perform, 8 oz. PowerBar, Inc.	60	0	16	13	0	0	Glucose, fructose, maltodextrin	BCAAs, N-Acetyl cysteine, glutamine, chromium, magnesium, vitamin C, B_3, B_6, E, pantothenic acid
XLR8 30 ml with 28 oz. fluid (concentrate)	124	0	31	10	0	0	Glucose, fructose, glucose polymers	Glycerol, magnesium, sodium, potassium, calcium
Cytomax, 1 scoop Champion Nutrition (powder)	95	0	20	11	0	0	Maltodextrin, fructose, glucose	Sodium, potassium, vitamin C, amino acids
Ultrafuel, 8 oz. Twinlab	200	0	50	30	0	0	Glucose polymers, glucose, fructose	Vitamin C, B_1, B_2, B_3, B_6, biotin, pantothenic acid, potassium, magnesium, chromium
ProHydrator, 8 oz. Inter Nutria	0		0	0	0	0	n/a	Glycerol, potassium, sodium
Fruit drinks								
Vruit, 8.45 oz. American Soy Products	120	1	29	27	0	0	Apple/carrot juice blend and orange/veggie blend—100% juice	Vitamin C, A, shelf-life packaging

Type	Calories	Proteins	Carb*	Sugar	Fat	Fiber	Sugar Source	Extras
Fruit smoothies								
Hansen's Natural Fruit Juice Smoothie, 1 can	170–180	0–1	43–44	42–43	0	0	Fruit puree, high-fructose corn syrup	100% Vitamins A, C, E, B_2, B_3, B_6, 12, iron, taurine**
Hansen's Lite Fruit Juice Smoothie, 1 can	50	0	13	13	0	0	Fruit puree, aspartame	100% Vitamins A, C, E, calcium
Smoothie King 20 oz. Fruit Smoothie** Raspberry Sunrise	335	3	84	0	0	0	Turbinado, honey	Vitamins A, C, calcium, iron
Lifestyle beverages								
Hansen's Healthy Start Juices*, 1 serving	110–130	0–1	28–32	4–31	0	0	Fruit juice concentrate	Vitamins A, C, D, E, B_1, B_3, pantothenic acid, biotin, calcium, selenium, echinacea, grapeseed extract, hawthorn, gingko biloba, ginseng**
Hansen's Functionals** (carbonated), 1 can	110–120	0	31–32	29–32	0	0	High-fructose corn syrup, glucose	Vitamins A, C, E, B_2, B_3, B_6, B_{12}, creatine, taurine, glutamine, ginseng, St. John's wort, L-Tyrosine, kava kava, chamomile, L-carnitine, bee pollen, royal jelly, coenzyme Q, guarana, grape seed extract, selenium, echinacea, ginkgo biloba, guarana, schizandra berry**
SoBe**, 8 oz. South Beach Beverage Co.	120**	0	32	31	0	0	High-fructose corn syrup	Vitamins A, C, ginkgo biloba, ginseng, guarana, selenium, bee pollen, echinacea, St. John's wort, schizandra, arginine, yohimbe, creatine, taurine, proline+

Coffee drinks

Type	Calories	Proteins	Carb	Sugar	Fat	Sat. Fat	Fiber	Sugar Source	Extras
Westbrae, Coffee Beverage, 8 oz. Westbrae, Inc.	130	2	25	23	0	0		Cane juice	Potassium, sodium, calcium
Power Frappuccino, 12 oz. Starbucks (Tall)	290*	8	61	31	2.0	0		Maltodextrin	Vitamins A, B_1, B_2, B_3, C, D, E, folate, biotin, pantothenic acid, calcium
Grande Size 16 oz.	350	9	73	42	2.5	0		Maltodextrin	Same
Venti Size 20 oz.	410	10	86	52	3.0	0		Maltodextrin	Same

Type	Calories	Proteins	Carb	Sugar	Fat	Sat. Fat	Fiber	Sugar Source	Extras
Sport Shakes									
Balanced American Natural Snacks, Inc.	230	15	37	19	3	0.5	0	Dehydrated cane juice	Soy-based, all-natural, lactose-free, 25–50% vitamin-fortified
High Protein Balance	230	15	35	19	3	0.5	3	Same as above	Same as above
Diet Balance	180	10	34	28	1	0	3	Same as above	Same as above
Complete Pacific Foods	200	9	33	20	3	0	3	Cane juice sweetener	20–50% vitamin-fortified; Omega 3 source
Met-Rx, Total Nutrition Met-Rx, Inc.	240	38	19	3	2.5	1.5	3	Maltodextrin	40–100% vitamin-fortified
Met-Rx Ready-to-Drink	160	20	19	8	1	0	1	Brown rice syrup	130% C, 340% E

*Fruit juices and soft drinks usually have 10–11% carbohydrate concentration provided.
**Dependent on flavor and variety.
†List may be incomplete.

121

Bottoms Up

Before cooling off with a great big glass of your favorite thirst quencher, consider the following facts regarding your fluid needs.

▶ On a daily basis, consume at least a liter of water, and more when you're training. If you're bored with tap or bottled, try the flavored, sparkly kind. You can also have some fun and explore the shelves for a New Age drink, smoothie, or tea reviewed in the Fluid and Lifestyle Beverages table. With the variety of tastes, extra sugar energy, and perhaps some of the missing vitamins, minerals, and antioxidants from your food diet, a new exotic fruit blend might hit the spot.

▶ Caution: Read the label . . . Not only do the calories add up, but so does the sugar content. For instance, R. W. Knudsen's Simply Delicious Ginkgo Alert has eight servings of 120 calories in one 32-ounce container. Boy, did I stay awake, and not only from the ginkgo! With about seven teaspoons of sugar (28 grams) per 4-ounce cup, I drank 56 teaspoons of sugar and 960 calories in one sitting!

▶ If you're trying to lose weight or have any type of high or low blood sugar problems, watch the calorie and sugar content. Calculate the nutrients into your food diet. For most of the beverages, it would take the place of foods from the fruit group (see chapter 9), since fruits are primarily carbohydrates. For every 60-calorie serving, you spend one fruit. However, you don't get the fiber and some of the nutrients from the real foods from that group.

▶ For lifestyle beverages, use caution with the extra vitamins, minerals, and herbs. Just like supplements, too much of a good thing is just too much (see chapter 8). Evaluate the extras according to your personal needs and present food diet.

▶ If you're a professional athlete, read the label. Some contain illegal herbs for international competition. Either way, you'll want to add Varro Tyler's books to your library for the best and most thorough review of herbs. Two of them are *Herbs of Choice* and *The Honest Herbal,* excellent resources on herbs, efficacy, and research.

▶ Fluid and Lifestyles Beverages ◀
Herbs and Supplements Chart

INGREDIENT/PURPOSE	EFFECTIVENESS/SAFETY
Herbs	
Echinacea: immune stimulant, wound healer; may shorten duration and frequency of common cold, also supportive treatment of recurrent infections of upper respiratory tract and lower urinary tract; increases white blood cells and spleen cells	Caution with individuals suffering from systemic diseases such as TB or MS, also collagen disorders, HIV; side effects—do not use for more than an 8-week period
Ephedra (Ma Huang): a.k.a. sea grape, yellow horse, Mormon Tea, and sida cordifolia; .5 mg/kg body weight, 300 mg total; used for one week or less, may clear up respiratory infections and congestion associated with asthma; CNS stimulant; BANNED by the IOC and NCAA	Similar to amphetamines—increases heart rate and blood pressure, may cause palpitations, tachycardia, arrhythmia, headaches, nausea, vomiting, restlessness, irritability, seizures, and death . . . not advised
Ginkgo Biloba: enhances cerebral blood flow, functions as "free-radical" scavenger (see chapter 7); 120–240 mg/day of standardized extract taken over 2–3 doses recommended for dementia	May cause GI disturbance, dizziness, headache, heart palpitations, and skin rashes; not to be consumed by those on blood thinners or individuals hypersensitive to poison ivy, cashews, or mangos
Ginseng: ancient tonic from China and Russia, a.k.a. "adaptogen"; Korean Panax Ginseng most desirable; increases resistance to chemical, physical, and biological stress; may build general vitality, including physical and mental capacities	No serious adverse effects; most common are nervousness and excitation; possible diarrhea and hypoglycemia
Guarana: central nervous system stimulant; high caffeine content	Acts like caffeine; added to Coca-Cola in Brazil; nervousness, insomnia, rapid and irregular heartbeats, elevated sugar, cholesterol levels, stomach acid, and heartburn may result in those sensitive
Hawthorn: dilates blood vessels, especially heart; also reduces peripheral resistance lowering blood pressure. Has flavonoids, a phytochemical that may produce sedative effects on CNS	Effective and safe in healthy individuals

INGREDIENT/PURPOSE

EFFECTIVENESS/SAFETY

Schizandra: adaptogen—may increase resistance to disease and stress, increase immunity. May act as antioxidant, protect liver, and stimulate energy

Inconclusive results; no known side effects

St. John's Wort: named after John the Baptist because flowers abundant on his birthday, June 24. Used for insomnia, gastritis, inflammation, and hemorrhoids externally. Best known as antidepressant. Acts as MAO inhibitor and serotonin uptake blocker; 300 mg dry extract recommended for mildly depressed individuals only

Dermatitis and inflammation to mucous membranes when exposed to sunlight; may increase duration and intensity of migraine headaches; do not take with caffeine or guarana-containing foods and beverages

Yohimbé: aphrodisiac, dilates skin blood vessels and lowers blood pressure, MAO inhibitor

Do not take with blood pressure meds, diet pills, nasal decongestants, or MAO inhibitors; do not take with tyramine-containing foods, e.g., cheese, wine, liver; high doses linked to weakness and paralysis; persons with heart, liver, or kidney disease should not consume this herb

Supplements

A-Acetyl Cysteine (NAC): antioxidant, derivative of amino acid cysteine; used successfully as an antidote for acetaminophen toxicity; precursor of GSH, another antioxidant; may decrease severity and length of flulike symptoms; may reduce duration and incidence of bronchitis

Mild side effects if any—nausea and skin rash

Bee pollen: not necessarily from bees; pollens are composed of polysaccharides (50%), sugar (4–10%), fats, and protein; maybe Vitamin C and carotenoids

Not safe; can cause severe allergic response in sensitive individuals, diarrhea, asthma attacks. Not found to be therapeutic

Branched chain amino acids (BCAAs): isoleucine, leucine, and valine may have a role in preventing central nervous system fatigue in exercise, since they compete with tryptophan to the brain and prolonged exercise increases tryptophan-to-BCAA ratio and allows tryptophan to increase brain levels of serotonin and cause fatigue; may also prevent protein breakdown in muscles and energy source during prolonged exercise

Inconclusive; high doses can lead to increased blood ammonia levels, which can lead to fatigue, impair water absorption, and cause GI distress; may cause displacement of other amino acids

INGREDIENT/PURPOSE

Carnitine: vitaminlike compound isolated from meat products, essential for transferring fatty acids; to the mitochondria to be used for energy; also converts branched chain amino acid analogues during fasting, starvation, and exercise

Ciwujia: marketed under brand name Endurox; dose is 9–27 grams per day and may fight fatigue and boost immune system; may also decrease lactic acid levels and increase use of energy from fat

Chromium Picolate: helps facilitate the uptake of sugar by the cells and helps insulin control blood sugar; regulates protein synthesis by promoting amino acid uptake by cells

Glutamine: important amino acid involved with the immune system; energy source for muscle, since it converts to alanine and is used as glucose; depleted during stress and exercise, especially overtraining syndrome. Pre-exercise glutamine levels dependent on intensity and duration of training. Depletion causes increased susceptibility to infection

Green Tea Polyphenols: potent antioxidant compounds; may increase activity of antioxidant enzymes and inhibit formation of nitrosamines from high-nitrite foods at mealtime

Royal Jelly: produced by bees, causes queen bee to become fertile; increased fertility not proven in humans; contains protein, carbohydrates, fatty acids, and B vitamins; used for rejuvenating the skin

EFFECTIVENESS/SAFETY

Use only drink products containing L-carnitine; the D form may produce muscle pain and loss of muscle function (and energy)

Appears to be safe; further research needed

Questionable safety with picolinate chelator; picolinic acid helps facilitate chromium absorption but may cause damage to DNA; better without if supplemented. More research is needed

Safe in doses not to exceed .57 grams glutamine/kg/bw/day or about 30 grams/day in three doses of 10 grams

Safe and recommended

May cause asthma attacks, skin irritation—not advised

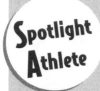

Spotlight Athlete

Ben Richardson
World-class Laser sailor

Age: 22

4 years semivegetarian (vegan at times)

Reason for becoming vegetarian: "Weight management."

Advantages of being vegetarian: "Helps maintain ideal weight for sport."

Challenges to being vegetarian: "Was vegan for one and one half years until a ten-day trip with no protein sources available led me to eat chicken and fish again."

Supplements: chromium and creatine

Favorite prerace meal: Ben's "Smooth Sailing" Laser Oatmeal (chapter 3, page 51) and 32 oz water

Favorite snacks: Balance Bar or ice cream

Favorite one-pot meal: tortilla sandwich

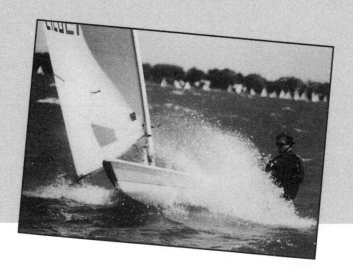

Spotlight Athlete

Charlene Wong Williams
Olympic and professional figure skater

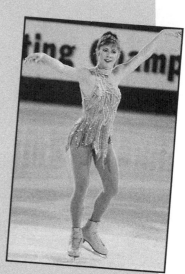

▷ *Age:* 32

▷ 10 years primarily vegan vegetarian

▷ *Reason for becoming vegetarian:* "Wanted to feel better, healthier and improve my appearance (weight).
I also or should I especially say I wanted to observe the relationship between food, mood, and cravings."

▷ *Advantages of being vegetarian:* "In order to be healthy and vegetarian, I believe it's even more important to make informed food choices than when not a veggie. This in turn has a profound effect on your well-being and enhances your performance."

▷ *Challenges to being vegetarian:* "It takes a commitment to do a little extra for planning meals, especially when traveling."

▷ *Alcohol:* none

▷ *Supplements:* See Charlene's Skating Supplement (pages 169–170)

▷ *Favorite pre-event meal depends on time of day and season:*
mornings, winter or fall—hot cereal or rice, whole-grain toast, beans or nut butter, rice milk, weak black tea; spring and summer—whole-grain bread, fruit spread and nut butter, juice, tea. Afternoons, fall or winter—soup, tempeh and rice, leafy greens, fruit juice, green tea; spring or summer—salad, tofu/veggie stir-fry, fruit compote, green tea.

▷ *Favorite snacks:* edamame (boiled soybeans in husk), regular popcorn, kabocha squash, root veggie or corn chips, radishes, ginger/shoyu tea with kuzu

▷ *Favorite one-pot meal:* Charlene's Triple Axel Veggie Surprise (page 90)

Dave Scott's Pre-Sport Shake

Makes 1 serving

1 tbs peanut butter, smooth

$\frac{1}{2}$ cup plain soy yogurt

1 banana

4 fresh large strawberries

$\frac{1}{2}$ cup orange juice

Triathlon consumption: Blend. Drink. Race.

▶ Nutrients per serving: 363 calories, 13 grams protein, 62 grams carbohydrates, 9 grams fat, 2 grams saturated fat, 4 grams monounsaturated fat, 2.5 grams linoleic fat, 42 grams sugar, 7 grams fiber

▶ Dietary composition: 14% protein, 64% carbohydrates, 22% fat

▶ VSNG food servings: 1 milk, 3½ fruits, ½ protein, 1 fat*

▶ Good source of vitamin B_6, C, folate, potassium; moderate source of vitamin B_2, B_3, B_{12}, K, pantothenic acid, calcium, phosphorus, magnesium, manganese

*Food fitness note: You can save on fat grams by using fat-free soy yogurt. It might also be tasty with vanilla-flavored yogurt.

7

The Athlete's Lab: Vitamins, Minerals, and Phytochemicals

CRAIG HEATH is a professional figure skater and four-time American and Canadian gold medalist. At age 31, he performs in ten to twelve Disney on Ice shows per week while training for competition. He credits his 16 years as a vegetarian for helping him "stay on top by eating right all the time."

Craig is quick to tell you that he is always told how young he looks. As a result, he's able to play younger parts in ice performances. Craig is always full of energy and "abundant stamina," which is critical for excelling in figure skating. His daily diet consists of cereal, fruit, soy milk, beans, greens, pasta, and rice or potato. The only challenge he faces is being on the road ten to eleven months a year without a traditional kitchen to prepare his favorite dishes, particularly Heath's Skating Mexican Fiesta Meal (on page 95 of chapter 5).

Craig's favorite pre-event high-carb meal is pasta with red sauce, water, and a sport drink. He snacks on nutrient-dense peanut butter and jelly, rice cakes, and even some health-nut cookies. Always looking for new ways to get energy and strength, "I'm on a lifetime journey in a healthy direction." Regardless of the high nutritional quality of his alcohol-free diet, Craig supplements his intake with more than ten vitamins a day, two energy drinks, and green tea.

Vitamin and Mineral Warmup

Fine-tuning an eating program with vitamins, minerals, and phyto-chemicals reminds me of the sport of figure skating. While inter-viewing skaters like Craig, Charlene, and others, as I recall watching these champions compete and perform, I marvel at their athletic abil-ities enhanced with the beauty and creativity of their dance.

This finely tuned sport can be compared to the role that vitamins, minerals, and phytochemicals play in the body. Even though carbo-hydrates, proteins, and fats create adenosine triphosphate (ATP) energy for the working muscle, without vitamins and minerals, the body cannot use these fuels effectively, particularly under stress. Without a consistent intake of the right balance of these fuel facilita-tors and cell protectors, the body compromises the way it uses energy. Similarly, without the beauty of dance movement with skat-ing performance, it's just skating.

The Science

Even though vitamins and minerals do not give energy, they are the links and regulators of energy-producing and muscle-building path-ways. When compared to the amount of grams needed for fats, pro-tein, and carbohydrates, hundredths of those amounts are needed for vitamins and minerals.

Vitamins are defined as a group of unrelated "organic" compounds essential to the body in small amounts. There are the fat-soluble vita-mins, A, D, E, and K, and the water-soluble vitamins, the B's and C. This property determines how they are absorbed, transported, excreted, and stored in the body.

Digestion and Absorption

About 40 to 90% of ingested vitamins are absorbed primarily in the small intestine. Fat-soluble vitamins are absorbed with dietary fat, trav-eling through the lymphatic system to reach the bloodstream. Water-soluble vitamins are transported in blood, bound to specific carrier proteins. Therefore, a protein deficiency can potentially cause a sec-ondary deficiency of many vitamins.

Once inside the body, vitamins must be transported to the cells where they are needed. Since many vitamins are absorbed in a provitamin form, they need to become active before they can be used. The rate and amount of provitamin conversion will determine the amount available to the body. The ability to store and secrete these vitamins will also regulate the amount available for use.

Requirements

To determine vitamin and mineral requirements, absorption, transport, metabolism, storage, and excretion must be considered. Studies used to determine dietary needs are

- ▶ Depletion-repletion studies: diets deficient in the vitamin/mineral are fed until deficiency symptoms disappear.
- ▶ Nutrient balance studies: compare intake to excretion.
- ▶ Animal studies: extrapolate information gathered from experiments with rats, mice, monkeys, or other animals.
- ▶ Epidemiological studies: requirements based on population observations of nutrient status in relation to dietary intake. These studies are used to determine the Recommended Dietary Allowances (RDAs).

The Recommended Dietary Allowances (RDAs) are defined as the recommended safe and adequate average daily intakes that will meet the known nutrient needs of the majority of individuals. The RDAs were originally developed in 1940 by the Food and Nutrition Board of the National Research Council at the request of the government. They have been updated about every 10 years under the guidance of a diverse group of scientific experts to reflect the latest information in the most recent scientific literature.

The RDAs include recommendations for eleven vitamins and seven minerals, protein (grams daily) and energy (calories). The vitamins include A, C, D, E, K, B_1, B_2, B_3, B_6, B_{12}, and folate; the minerals are calcium, phosphorous, iron, zinc, iodine, and selenium. In the RDA's ninth edition, a category called the Estimated Safe and Adequate Daily Dietary Intakes (ESADDI) for two additional vitamins and eight minerals was established. These vitamins and minerals have sufficient data to estimate a range of requirements, but insufficient information for establishing a RDA. They include biotin, pantothenic acid, chromium, molybdenum, copper, manganese, fluoride, sodium, chloride, and potassium.

The Food and Drug Administration (FDA) has used the RDAs for food labeling as the U.S. RDAs. The U.S. RDAs were initially set in 1973 for protein and nineteen vitamins and minerals based on the maximum amount of each nutrient needed for any adult age group. The U.S. RDAs have recently been replaced by the Reference Daily Intakes (RDIs). The RDIs are the highest RDA for each nutrient to ensure that all individuals are covered. Since they were compiled in 1968 to use for the 1973 U.S. RDAs, they are outdated and impose limitations.

Do the RDAs Meet the Needs of Athletes?

The RDAs were never intended to meet minimal requirements or optimal intakes. Strenuous physical activity is described as a condition that may require adjustment in the application of the RDAs since "increased activity increases the need for energy and some nutrients."

Additional research indicates that work capacity, oxygen consumption, and other measures of physical performance of individuals, including athletes, are affected by deficiency or borderline deficiency of specific vitamins or essential trace elements. However, if the athlete consumes substantial daily calories from nutritious plant-based sources, the diet will meet or exceed the RDAs and ESADDIs, as in the case of most of the athletes in this book.

This chapter will provide an overview of the vitamins, minerals, function, food sources, and daily recommended amounts. Chapter 8 will address the issue of supplementation, for athletes who demonstrate adequate status may benefit from additional amounts for peak performance.

Water-Soluble Vitamin Functions and Plant-Based Sources

The B Vitamins

The B vitamins are special to all athletes. B vitamins work in every cell, but this accounts for less than 1/1000th of what they do. B vitamins are part of one or more coenzymes that make it possible for the body's chemicals to work. A coenzyme is a small molecule that combines with an enzyme (made from proteins) to make the enzymes active. They also help the body release energy from carbohydrates, proteins, and fats. Therefore, deficiencies of any B vitamin can interfere with energy metabolism and affects all cells in the body.

The unique quality of B vitamins is that needs are determined individually. For thiamin (B_1), riboflavin (B_2), and niacin (B_3), recommendations are proportional to energy intake. For pyridoxine (B_6), needs are based on protein intake.

Since the best sources of B vitamins are animal products, vegetarian athletes need to meet their needs through unprocessed and/or whole grains. Beans and other "brown" foods (remember "b" in brown for the B vitamins) will also work. Craig and most of the other athletes have no trouble getting enough B's when consuming enough nutritious foods such as beans, peas, whole wheat bread, spinach, mushrooms, and asparagus. Sport bars, sport drinks such as the new Perform by PowerBar, sport shakes such as Balanced and Complete, and soy milks are also fortified with B vitamins.

Needs for these vitamins also increase proportionally with energy expenditure. That means that the plant-based athlete needs to consume extra portions of B-vitamin-rich food when increasing physical exercise.

Non-B Vitamins and Other Substances

Inositol, lipoic acid, and choline are sometimes called B vitamins. They are actually nonvitamins because they are not considered essential. Like the B vitamins, they serve as coenzymes in metabolism. Other substances sometimes called vitamins include para-aminobenzoic acid (PABA), bioflavinoids, and ubiquinone (coenzyme Q) because they are needed for growth by bacteria or other life. Vitamins B_{15} (pangamic acid), B_{17} (laetrile), and B_t (carnitine) have also been inaccurately called B vitamins. With the exception of carnitine, they are not necessary for health and are not considered vitamins.

Vitamin C

Along with the B's, the active forms of vitamin C act as a coenzyme or cofactor involved in the oxidation of food and energy production.

One active form, ascorbic acid, is also involved with

▶ collagen and hormone synthesis

▶ building the immune system

▶ enhancing iron absorption

▶ regenerating vitamin E and also serving as an antioxidant

Vitamin C is one of the most widely studied vitamins in relation to sport performance and exercise. In deficient states, the lack of collagen production can affect cartilage, tendons, ligaments, and other connective tissues. Also, since vitamin C is needed to make carnitine, which is in turn necessary for fatty acid transportation into the mitochondria, energy would be compromised.

Some other limitations imposed by deficiency include lack of energy due to inability to synthesize the stress hormone cortisol, the transport of iron, the metabolism of folic acid, and the inability to regenerate vitamin E for antioxidant purposes. For the athlete, these deficiencies can collectively result in poor injury healing, increased bruising, anemia, fatigue, muscular weakness, pain, and anorexia.

Vitamin C foods are the easiest ones to include for the vegetarian athlete because fruits and vegetables are the best sources. Orange juice, broccoli, cantaloupe, brussels sprouts, green pepper, tomatoes, and potatoes are all excellent choices.

Because the water-soluble vitamins are transported in body fluids and not stored, they need to be consumed daily. Taken in excess, they are excreted in the urine. However, some, such as niacin and pyridoxine, may have toxic effects.

Fat-Soluble Vitamins and Plant-Based Sources

The fat-soluble vitamins A, D, E, and K are found in the fats and oils of food. Like fat, they require bile (the fat emulsifier) for absorption. They are stored in body fat and the liver until the body needs them for a variety of important uses. Unlike the water-soluble vitamins, one can survive for weeks without an abundance of fat-soluble, vitamin-rich sources and avoid deficiency. However, consistently low intakes

▶ The Water-Soluble Vitamins ◀

VITAMIN	RDA	DEFICIENCIES	PLANT-BASED FOOD SOURCES
B_1, Thiamin	1.1–1.5 mg	Weakness, tingling, abnormal heart rhythms, edema	Seeds, black beans, green peas, watermelon, oatmeal, baked potato
B_2, Riboflavin	1.3–1.7 mg	Inflammation of mouth and tongue, cracks in corners of mouth	Spinach, mushrooms, enriched grains, soy products
B_3, Niacin	15–19 mg	Skin problems, diarrhea, dementia, dizziness	Enriched grains, peanuts, mushrooms, baked potato
B_6, Pyridoxine	1.6–2.0 mg	Headache, nausea, anemia, muscle twitching, skin rashes	Baked potato, watermelon, banana, spinach, navy beans, broccoli
B_{12}, Cobalamin	2 mcg	Pernicious anemia, poor nerve function, fatigue	Fortified products—cereals, breads, Red Star brand nutritional yeast
Folic Acid	180–200 mcg	Anemia, tongue inflammation, diarrhea, frequent infections	Spinach, turnip greens, lima beans, beets, asparagus, broccoli, orange juice, winter squash, cantaloupe, seeds
Pantothenic Acid	4–7 mcg	Fatigue, rash, insomnia	Whole grains, legumes
Biotin	30–100 mcg	Skin problems, nausea, depression, muscle pain	Synthesized in gut; fortified foods
Vitamin C	60 mg	Poor wound healing, bleeding gums	Orange juice, broccoli, cantaloupe, brussels sprouts, green pepper, tomatoes and juice, baked potato

and foods that may affect absorption, for example, fat substitutes like Olestra (see chapter 5) are two factors that may increase the risk of deficiency.

Fat-soluble vitamins function more like hormones than the water-soluble B's and C do. Each plays a specific and unique role in the body. Vitamins A and D direct cells to convert one substance to another.

Vitamin E prevents oxidative destruction of tissues. Vitamin K is necessary for blood to clot.

Vitamin A

Vitamin A is essential for vision, growth, and reproduction. It is derived from a group of compounds called carotenoids. Beta-carotene is the vitamin A precursor, an orange pigment found in plants. Retinol is one of the active forms of vitamin A, made from beta-carotene and stored in the liver. When beta-carotene is converted in the body to retinol, losses occur. That is why vitamin A amounts on food labels and some tables are reflected in retinol equivalents (RE) to provide the actual amount of retinol available after conversion.

One retinol equivalent equals

- 1 microgram retinol
- 6 micrograms beta-carotene
- 12 micrograms other carotenoid vitamin A precursors
- 3.33 International Units (IU) vitamin A activity from retinol (some food tables use this unit)
- 10 IU vitamin A activity from beta-carotene
- 20 IU vitamin A activity from other carotenoid vitamin A precursors

Vegetarians have no problems getting enough vitamin A from carrots, sweet potatoes, spinach, butternut squash, cantaloupe, broccoli, fortified milk, and soy milk. For athletes, vitamin A serves as an antioxidant to protect the body from excessive free radical production (see free radical box). It is possible that as an antioxidant, vitamin A is required for the increased metabolism for exercise and for tissue repair. However, research has not examined vitamin A without other antioxidants such as vitamin C and E, which appear to have the strongest antioxidant relationship in athletes.

Excessive vitamin A intakes can be toxic. Research shows that individuals who are heavy smokers and drinkers are at greater risk for lung cancer and heart disease from excessive amounts. However, the benign toxicity of eating too many carrots and turning yellow under the fat pads of the skin in the hands and feet is not a concern.

Free Radicals

Free radicals are loose oxygen particles formed as a natural part of metabolism. These highly reactive oxygen molecules attach themselves to the body's DNA and RNA molecules. The result can be tissue damage and destruction—prerequisites for cancer, heart disease, autoimmune diseases, and diabetes.

Athletes run the risk of increased free radical production because physical activity

- causes use of about 10 to 20 times more oxygen than non-activity
- increases metabolism and lactic acid production
- elevates pre- and postexercise hemoglobin oxidation
- increases exercise-induced hyperthermia
- causes a transient lack of oxygen and reoxygenation of joints and muscles during exercise

When compounded with the effects of training in sunlight, radiation, air pollution, and smoke, the damage could be worse since the body only has a limited store of antioxidants to defend itself. Vitamins A, E, and C, selenium, and some phytochemicals have been found to be powerful natural antioxidant substances.

Vitamin D

Vitamin D is different from other vitamins and minerals because in addition to food sources, it can be synthesized in the body through sunlight. When the sun shines on the cholesterol component of skin, it is transformed into a vitamin D precursor and absorbed directly into the blood.

The primary role of vitamin D is to maintain calcium and phosphorus balance in the body in order to maintain bone formation and maintenance, neuromuscular function, and other cellular processes. There is very little research on its specific role in sports other than general health maintenance.

Although vegetarian athletes do not routinely include traditional sources of Vitamin D, found in milk, liver, eggs, and fish, most are generally exposed to sunlight during training and competition, consume fortified foods such as sport bars, sport shakes, and soy milks, or take a supplement to meet their needs.

Vitamin E

Vitamin E, known as the tocopherol group of vitamins, has been found to be the most effective natural antioxidant, playing a critical role in preventing heart disease and certain types of cancer. Alpha tocopherol, the most common form, protects beta carotene and spares selenium, the mineral antioxidant. By protecting the cells of the body, vitamin E maintains the integrity of red blood cells, nervous tissue, and the immune system. Athletes are rarely deficient in vitamin E. However, research has looked at the possible role it may play in muscle damage and recovery after exercise.

Vegetable oils, sunflower seeds, nuts, whole grains, and wheat germ are good food sources. Fortified cereals, sport bars, shakes, and drinks such as Perform have also included vitamin E in their formulas.

Vitamin K

Vitamin K is responsible for synthesizing four proteins involved with blood clotting. It is used rapidly by the body and needs to be constantly supplied for injuries, normal daily living wear and tear, and preventing blood loss. Since there is no clear association with vitamin K and exercise, athletes need to consume the same amounts of vitamin K as nonexercising individuals.

The form of vitamin K found in plants is phylloquinone. The best food sources are leafy greens, broccoli, brussels sprouts, and kale. The bacteria in the gastrointestinal tract produce some vitamin K, so deficiency is rarely a problem.

The functions, RDAs, and best plant-based food sources for the fat-soluble vitamins are summarized in the fat-soluble vitamins chart.

▶ The Fat-Soluble Vitamins ◀

VITAMIN	RDA	DEFICIENCIES	PLANT-BASED FOOD SOURCES
A	800–1000 RE	Dry skin, night blindness	Carrots, greens, sweet potato, butternut squash, cantaloupe, fortified milks
D	5 mcg	Bone softness	Through sunlight; fortified margarine, milks, and soy beverages
E	8–10 TE*	Blood cell breakdown, nerve damage, anemia, weakness, leg cramps	Vegetable oils, leafy greens, nuts, seeds, sweet potatoes, wheat germ
K	65–80 mcg	Hemorrhage	Synthesized in intestinal tract, cabbage-type vegetables, leafy greens

*.74 alpha tocopherol equivalents (TE) = 1 mg alpha tocopherol = 1 IU Vitamin E

Major Minerals

The dietary elements required by the body in the greatest amounts are carbon, hydrogen, oxygen, and nitrogen. The next group of important food elements is the major minerals—calcium, phosphorus, magnesium, sodium, chloride, potassium, and sulfur. The human body is composed of approximately 4% of these and fourteen other minerals. They are needed by the body in amounts greater than 100 mg per day.

Minerals work with enzymes to facilitate chemical reactions and also contribute to the body's structural components. Many minerals are important in energy production, while other minerals called electrolytes (sodium, potassium, and chloride) are responsible for muscle contraction, nerve conduction, and fluid balance. Calcium, phosphorus, and magnesium found primarily in bone help to maintain bone density and normal nerve and muscle contractions. Sulfur is present in all proteins, insulin, chondroitin sulfate in bone and cartilage, and the vitamins biotin and thiamin. Sulfur influences the rigidity of the proteins found in skin, nails, and hair. An overview of the major minerals can be found below.

▶ The Major Minerals ◀

MINERAL	RDA	DEFICIENCIES	PLANT-BASED FOOD SOURCES
Calcium	1200 mg	Risk for osteoporosis	Tofu, greens, legumes, blackstrap molasses, sea vegetables, hiziki, quinoa, buckwheat, broccoli, bok choy, tofu made w/calcium
Phosphorus	1200 mg	Bone loss, weakness, poor appetite	Cereals and baked goods
Magnesium	280 mg females, 350 mg males	Nausea, vomiting, weakness, heat changes	Nuts, legumes, whole grains, dark greens,chocolate, and cocoa
Sodium	500 mg min., 2400 mg max.	Muscle cramps	Table salt, sea salt, soy sauce, natural "fast foods," soy cheeses, sport drinks
Chloride	750–3400 mg	Cramps, mental apathy, loss of appetite	Sport drinks, table salt, soy sauce, natural "fast foods," soy cheeses
Potassium	1600– 3500 mg	Dehydration, irregular heartbeat, fatigue, muscle cramps	Fruits, vegetables, grains, legumes, sport drinks
Sulfur	None specified	Protein deficiency occurs first	All protein-containing foods

Trace Minerals

The trace minerals are found in smaller quantities in the body than the major minerals. The trace minerals are defined as elements with estimated dietary requirements of less than 100 mg per day. Over the last 25 years, research has suggested that they are essential for health and life. One or more of the trace minerals has been shown to play a role in the development of heart disease, osteoporosis, osteoarthritis, and hypertension. These trace minerals are iron, fluoride, zinc, copper, silicon, vanadium, tin, nickel, selenium, manganese, iodine, molybdenum, chromium, and cobalt.

Trace elements are found in both plant and animal sources. The trace mineral contents of plants vary because soil concentrations of minerals vary according to region and can be affected by soil and water contamination. Once in the body, the bioavailability of trace minerals can be affected by an individual's health, nutritional status, and composition of the total diet.

The amount of trace minerals available to the body's tissues is dependent on the delivery from transporting proteins to specific tissue sites, hormone regulation, and the interaction between other minerals and components of the diet. These components, known as phytates, oxalates, and tannins (see chapter 8), are found in fresh vegetables and tea and can bind the minerals and leave them unavailable for the body. All of these complexities and effects on individual needs have made it difficult to determine specific requirements.

Some ultra-trace minerals, known to be essential for animals but yet to be determined for humans, are boron, arsenic, cadmium, lead, lithium, aluminum, bromine, rubidium, and tin. Since those already in the body can meet requirements for months or years, balance studies are difficult to conduct. Researchers would need to control the environment and total diet, since everything that comes in contact with the individual can have an impact on the small amounts required by the body.

Trace element toxicity is also a concern. Environmental pollution such as chipped lead paint, soil and air contamination, and excessive supplementation can compromise the bioavailability of the trace minerals, create an imbalance, and interfere with critical health functions. A summary of the trace minerals and some of the ultra-trace minerals can be found on pages 142 and 143.

▶ Trace Minerals ◀

MINERAL	RDA	DEFICIENCIES	PLANT-BASED FOOD SOURCES
Iron	10–15 mg	Anemia, weakness, lethargy	Whole or enriched grains, dried fruits, legumes, leafy greens, tofu, fermented miso, tempeh, soy sauce, blackstrap molasses, brewer's yeast
Fluoride	1.5–4.0 mg	Cavities	Fluoridated water, tea, toothpaste
Zinc	12–15 mg	Poor skin, poor immune system, taste loss	Nuts, seeds, whole grains, tofu, tempeh
Copper	1.5–3.0 mg	Anemia	Nuts, seeds
Silicon	5–20 mg*	Bone and connective tissue abnormalities (animals)	Whole grains and root vegetables
Vanadium	10 mcg	Thyroid changes	Mushrooms, parsley, dill seed, black pepper
Nickel	60–260 mcg	Decreased blood sugars, impaired reproduction, depressed growth (animal studies)	Chocolate, nuts, legumes and dried beans, peas, whole grains
Selenium	55–70 mcg	Muscle pain and weakness	Grains and vegetables dependent on soil conditions
Manganese	2–5 mg	Impaired growth, skeletal abnormalities, depressed reproduction, defects in fat metabolism	Unrefined cereals, nuts, leafy greens
Iodine	150 mcg	Depressed thyroid	Iodized salt, plants grown in iodized soil
Molybdenum	75–250 mcg	Impaired reproduction	Milk and milk products, legumes, cereal and baked goods, grains and legumes

MINERAL	RDA	DEFICIENCIES	PLANT-BASED FOOD SOURCES
Chromium	50–200 mcg	Impaired glucose metabolism	Grains, nuts, brewer's yeast
Cobalt	No RDA	B12-related anemia	Vegetables, whole grains
Boron	.5–3.1 mg avg. daily intake	Deficiency increases urinary excretion of calcium and magnesium and steroid hormones	Noncitrus fruits, nuts, legumes, cider, wine, beer, greens
Arsenic	12–15 mcg	Reproduction and growth problems	Grains and cereals

*There is no RDA or ESADDI for silicon; however, this is an estimated recommended range for requirement.

Minerals and Sports

Whether or not the RDA mineral amounts for athletes are adequate is unknown. Studies have shown that certain minerals are lost from the body during exercise by increased urination or sweating. For many, there is also no adequate routine biochemical method for assessing the status. However, one of the minerals with the longest and best-described history in sports that possesses a practical and accurate biochemical test is iron. This mineral or the lack of it has been found to have an impact on sports performance.

Iron is needed in greater amounts for athletes because exercise stimulates the production of red blood cells. Iron is needed for the hemoglobin portion of the cell. Iron is also needed for the muscle protein myglobin and iron-containing proteins needed for ATP energy production. Endurance and VO2max are reduced when an athlete is anemic. Performance improves when hemoglobin levels rise.

Iron deficiency is the most common single nutrient deficiency disease in the world, affecting approximately 15% of the population. Although exercise does not increase the risk for nutritional deficiencies, low iron status is common in athletes. This is due to a redistribution of iron from training. Adolescent and female athletes are at the greatest risk due to monthly blood losses and poor eating habits; however, the incidence of iron deficiency anemia in these groups is not higher than in nonathletic American females.

Deficiencies have also been a concern for the vegetarian athletes, since they do not consume the most readily available heme form of iron. Heme iron from meat has a 5 to 35% absorption rate from a single meal when compared to that of non-heme plant-based iron, 2 to 20%. Non-heme iron in plant foods is more sensitive to inhibitors and enhancers of absorption. Dietary fortification of sport bars, shakes, and cereals and the addition of beans, peas, dried fruits, whole and enriched grains, and blackstrap molasses help vegetarian athletes meet a greater percentage of their needs. Consuming these foods with a vitamin C-rich beverage or food enhances absorption. The athletes in this book have no problems meeting their daily iron needs as a result of their finely tuned, iron-rich vegetarian diets.

Sports Anemia

One of the earliest adaptations to regular aerobic exercise is the expansion of the blood plasma. As a result, endurance athletes tend to have lower hemoglobin concentrations than the general population. Sports anemia, also called dilutional pseudoanemia, which mimics low hemoglobin anemia, is considered a beneficial adaptation to exercise.

When an athlete continues on an exercise program, repeated muscle contractions during daily training can reduce the blood volume by as much as 10 to 20%. Much of the fluid lost in sweat comes from the blood. To compensate for this, the body releases hormones, which help conserve water and salt. As a result, blood volume expands, which dilutes red blood cells and lowers the concentration of hemoglobin. Despite the reduction of hemoglobin, more oxygen is delivered to the muscles and enhances performance.

True iron deficiency anemia, however, does not benefit the athlete. In the lab, if the hemoglobin is under 13 g/dl in a male or 11 g/dl in a female, a true anemia may be present. Signs of true iron deficiency anemia are a decline in performance; heavy, burning muscles; nausea; ice cravings; or cravings for cold, raw, crisp vegetables.

The Bone Minerals

Calcium, magnesium, and phosphorus are important to a wide variety of functions such as the mineralization of bone, maintaining muscle contraction and nerve stimulation, and serving as cofactors to many enzyme systems. Many athletes, especially females, consume less than adequate amounts of calcium and restrict calorie intakes to meet ideal competing weights, as in ballet, gymnastics, and long-distance running. The combination of calorie restriction and inadequate calcium can result in lack of menstruation and a decrease in bone mass. This leaves the athlete at risk for stress fractures and, later in life, osteoporosis. Vegetarian athletes can meet their calcium needs through low-fat dairy, fortified soy products, tofu, green vegetables, and legumes.

In addition to playing a role in carbohydrate metabolism and ATP-dependent reactions, magnesium interacts with calcium as an antagonist in muscle contraction. An excess of magnesium will inhibit bone calcification. Most studies report adequate dietary intakes of magnesium in athletes. However, performance can be compromised by diets high in refined foods, meat, and dairy.

Profuse sweating may cause magnesium losses in endurance athletes. Urinary excretion of magnesium has also been shown to increase after exercise. A vegetarian diet high in nuts, vegetables, whole grains, greens, and chocolate will meet the needs of most athletes.

All three minerals work together in the bone and blood. The blood concentration of calcium is also carefully maintained by the body for muscle contraction, nerve impulses, and blood clotting. If blood calcium levels drop, muscle cramps (inadvertent contractions—a condition called tetany) are a result. High blood phosphorus levels can also cause tetany by causing decreases of calcium in the blood.

Phosphorus is the second most abundant mineral in the body, 85% residing in the bones and teeth. It is critical to energy production as high-energy phosphates (see chapter 1) and as an acid-base buffer system to the body's cellular fluids. In this aspect, phosphate loading has been used as a successful technique for improving performance. It is also an important component of the group of fats called phospholipids (chapter 5).

Excesses of phosphorus can cause calcium excretion. Vegetarian athletes get adequate amounts from low-fat dairy, cereals, grains, nuts, and legumes.

Trace Minerals

The trace minerals that have received the most attention in sports and performance include iron and zinc. An overview of other trace minerals has been provided in the chart on page 142 and will be discussed in chapter 8. In addition to iron, discussed earlier, zinc has also received a considerable amount of attention in sports and demands extra attention for the plant-based athlete.

Zinc is a component of more than 100 enzymes involved in carbohydrate, protein, and fat metabolism. It plays an important role in tissue repair. It has also been shown to have antioxidant properties. Zinc losses from urine and sweat are a realistic concern for long-distance athletes. Although the athletes in this book have demonstrated adequate zinc intakes, it is a difficult mineral to assess because all foods have not been analyzed for zinc and the bioavailability of various foods differs.

Vegetarian diets generally contain adequate amounts of zinc from fortified grains, legumes, cheese, and peanut butter. However, due to fiber and phytates found in plant foods, zinc bioavailability may be compromised.

Phytochemicals

One of the hottest new topics in nutrition is phytochemicals. Although the health benefits of some of these potent substances were already known, the term used to describe some of the "phyto"-containing foods is new to the public.

Phytochemicals are nonessential nutrients found in thousands of plants (the origin of *phyto*). These compounds act as antioxidants, prevent the formation of cancer-causing nitrosamines in the digestive tract, block the enzymes that transform harmless chemicals into carcinogens that bind DNA, or neutralize carcinogens before they can bind to DNA. In fact, the National Cancer Institute has spent in excess of $20 million over the last five years researching the anticancer potential of plant foods. The inclusion of foods such as soy may even help to reduce cholesterol and triglycerides.

Consuming a diet rich in these plant foods is another "straw in the hat" for vegetarian diets. Foods and herbs with the highest anticancer potential are garlic, soybeans, cabbage, ginger, licorice, carrots, celery, cilantro, parsley, and parsnips. Modest levels of cancer-protective activity come from onions, flax, citrus, turmeric, cruciferous vegetables, tomatoes, peppers, brown rice, and whole wheat. Foods with mild activity are oats, barley, mint, rosemary, thyme, oregano, sage, basil, cucumber, cantaloupe, and berries.

Many of these foods and other phytochemical-rich foods have been included in the VSNG Peak Performance menus in chapters 9 and 10. Some of the best recipes are Stephens' No Horsing Around Veggie Plate, Hanners' Phyto Veggie Explosion, and Ruth's Ironwoman Pho, found in this chapter.

Although there has been no direct link from phytochemicals to sports success, perhaps some of the antioxidant properties can help with muscle recovery and performance. Perhaps it is other unidentified compounds in these foods that help with sport performance. And at a minimum, if eating these foods keeps the athlete healthier, then the athlete will perform better.

Some of the foods and their phytochemicals are listed in the table below.

▶ Phytochemicals and Health Benefits ◀

FOOD	PHYTOCHEMICAL	HEALTH BENEFIT
Garlic, onions, leeks, chives, shallots	Allylic sulfides	Reduce formation of nitrosamines; stimulate enzymes that detoxify carcinogens; may help with immune defenses
Hot peppers	Capsaicin	Prevents carcinogens from binding to DNA
Tomatoes (red pigment in other fruits and vegetables)	Lycopene	Antioxidant
Tomatoes, strawberries, and pineapple	Chlorogenic acid	Prevents carcinogenic molecules from binding to cells
Berries	Ellagic acid	Neutralizes carcinogens

FOOD	PHYTOCHEMICAL	HEALTH BENEFIT
Soy products	Flavonoids, phytosterols, genistein	Keep cancer-causing hormones from latching onto a cell-receptor site; prevent tumors from becoming solid; and possibly reduce cholesterol
Green and black tea	Flavonoids, polyphenols	Antioxidant
Avocados and watermelon	Glutathione	Antioxidant
Cruciferous vegetables	Indoles, sulforaphane	Stimulate enzymes that make estrogen less effective, possibly reducing cancer risk; may reduce stomach, colon, and breast cancers by triggering an enzyme to transport carcinogens out of the cell
Flaxseed	Lignins	May inhibit the growth of estrogen-stimulated breast cancer
Citrus fruits	Limonene	Shrinks tumors and prevents regrowth
Strawberries, pineapple, bell peppers	P-couramic, ferulic, and caffeic acids	Prevent binding of potentially carcinogenic molecules made during protein digestion
Grains	Phenols	Prevent carcinogens from reacting with target sites
Grains	Phytates and lignins	Deactivate potent hormones that stimulate tumor growth, especially in breast and prostate cancer; phytates suppress free radicals and act as antioxidants
Grapes	Resveratrol, flavonoids	Inhibit tumor growth; anti-inflammatory, anti-clotting properties
Grapes	Quercetin	Antioxidant
Tea	Tannins	Prevent carcinogens from reacting with target sites
Oranges, eggplant	Terpenes	Produce enzymes that deactivate carcinogens
Licorice root	Glycyrrhizen (and 400 other phytochemicals)	Enhances immunity by suppressing prostaglandins that are immune suppressors; blocks sex hormones, adds antioxidant action

Ruth's Ironwoman Pho

Makes 1 serving

$\frac{1}{2}$ cup brown long-grain rice, cooked

1 cup kale

$\frac{1}{2}$ cup broccoli

1 tsp miso

2 tbs yeast

1 tsp chili sauce (optional)

1 clove garlic

Mix in large serving bowl. Fill to top with water. Heat in microwave 4 minutes. Serve.

▶ Nutrients per serving: 244 calories, 14 grams protein, 43 grams carbohydrates, 2 grams fat, 4 grams sugar, $6\frac{1}{2}$ grams fiber

▶ Dietary composition: 22% protein, 70% carbohydrates, 7% fat

▶ VSNG food servings: $1\frac{1}{2}$ vegetables, 1.5 grains

▶ Good source of vitamin: A, C, B_1, B_2, B_3, B_6, E, K, folate, pantothenic acid, phosphorus, manganese; moderate source of potassium, magnesium, iron

▼

Stephens' No Horsing Around Veggie Plate

Makes 1 serving

———

1 cup mashed potato*
1 cup long-grain brown rice*
1 cup asparagus
1 cup broccoli

———

Prepare mashed potatoes, fresh or packaged (see author's food fitness note). Prepare rice (see food fitness note). Steam vegetables.

▶ Nutrients per serving: 466 calories, 18 grams protein, 97 grams carbohydrates, 4 grams fat, 1 gram monounsaturated fat, 1 gram linoleic fat

▶ Dietary composition: 15% protein, 78% carbohydrates, 7% fat

▶ VSNG food servings: 1^3/$_4$ vegetables, 5^1/$_2$ grains

▶ Good sources of vitamin B$_1$, B$_3$, B$_6$, A, C, E, K, folate, sodium, potassium, magnesium, selenium, phosphorus, manganese; moderate source of vitamin B$_2$, pantothenic acid, copper, zinc, iron

*Food Fitness Note: Barbara's has a quick, wholesome, chemical-free mashed potato mix. As always, brown rice is best!

Hanners' Phyto Veggie Explosion

Makes 2 servings

---

1 cup carrots, bias-cut
$\frac{1}{2}$ cup scallions, chopped
$\frac{1}{2}$ cup bok choy, stems and greens
3 fresh enoki or shiitake mushrooms
1 cup mung bean sprouts
1 cup snow peas

Oriental Phyto Fry Sauce
$\frac{1}{2}$ cup orange juice
$\frac{1}{2}$ cup lite soy sauce
1 tbs Dijon mustard
1 tbs rice vinegar
1 tbs honey
1 tbs water
$\frac{1}{2}$ tbs cornstarch or arrowroot
$\frac{1}{2}$ tbs garlic

Add all sauce ingredients in small saucepan. Bring to boil. Serve over steamed Phyto Veggies. Watch for explosion!

▶ Nutrients per serving (with sauce): 297 calories, 17 grams protein, 60 grams carbohydrates, 1 gram fat, 27 grams sugar, 6 grams fiber

▶ Dietary composition: 17% protein, 60% carbohydrates, 2% fat

▶ VSNG food servings: 2 vegetables, .5 fruit, 1.5 grains, . 5 protein

▶ Good source of vitamin A, C, K, folate, sodium, potassium; moderate source of vitamin B_1, B_2, B_3, B_6, pantothenic acid, phosphorus, magnesium, iron

Assessing Vitamin, Mineral, and Phytochemical Needs

One way to assess your need for potential missing vitamins, minerals, and phytochemical content of your diet is to compare your present diet with some of the information provided in this chapter. You can also find the spotlight vegetarian athlete's nutrition profile (Appendix A) that matches your sport or food intake. Take the profile and try to match it or use the Food Fitness Suggestions below the profile to improve your intake. This will give you a means of comparison and the approximate nutritional benefits and deficiencies of your diet.

If you want to get more personal, you can also use the dietary assessment form in Appendix B, calculate your nutrient needs using the formulas from chapters 1 through 5, and compare them to the specific calorie programs and menus in chapter 9. After you're finished, ask yourself the following questions:

Do you . . .

▶ Eat enough variety to potentially meet the RDAs for your vitamin or mineral needs?

▶ Eat enough food (calories) to help assimilate, transport, and metabolize the vitamin and/or mineral in question?

▶ Consume an abundance of products such as fiber, phytates, oxalates found in teas, and other foods that might bind your intake of vitamins and/or minerals?

▶ Prepare the foods you purchase in a timely fashion?

▶ Store the foods in hot, light, or exposed areas that may cause you to lose vitamins and minerals?

▶ Have special needs that may warrant additional vitamins and minerals from supplemental foods, shakes, or pills? (See chapter 8.)

▶ Have a medical problem, or are you pregnant, growing, drink alcohol, smoke, or take birth control or other medications that might validate the need for additional amounts?

▶ Believe your diet is chock full of energy and nutrients but continue to feel tired, lethargic, and depleted?

▶ Hear from your physician or registered dietitian (RD) that blood tests indicate a potential deficiency, like iron deficiency anemia?

▶ Find any of the signs and symptoms in the chart below that may indicate a subclinical deficiency?

▶ See a phytochemical-rich food that you can add, flavor, or season your food with to gain the potential health benefits?

After answering these questions, if you have any doubts that you might not be getting enough nutritious food, you can make simple changes to more of the best.

Some of these changes can include

▶ varying and purchasing new foods from each of the food groups in chapter 9. Try not to get into a food "jag," eating the same foods day after day. Select a variety of protein sources, grains, vegetables, fruits, and dairy products or alternatives from each food group.

▶ choosing at least five colors of food each day—white, brown, yellow/orange, green, and red—to ensure the best opportunity to consume all the vitamins and minerals.

▶ choosing the deepest colored foods, for example, deep-green versus light-green salads, or brown rice instead of white rice. Pigments from foods make our meals colorful and also provide valuable phytochemicals and antioxidants to make our meals rich with health benefits.

▶ eating the fresh foods you purchase within two days. Shop for those foods through your local farmer's market or Community Supported Agriculture (see chapter 10).

▶ storing all foods in dark containers in cool, dry locations. Invest in some airtight plastic containers!

▶ preparing foods with minimal liquids, cooking time, water and acids (juice, vinegar, tomatoes).

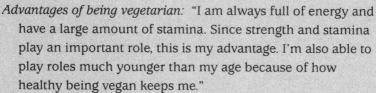

Craig Heath
Professional figure skater

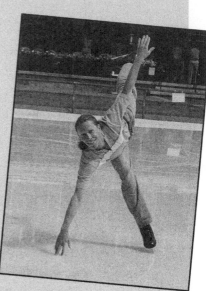

Age: 30

16 years vegetarian (vegan for the last 5 years)

Reason for becoming vegetarian: "When I was fourteen, I put it all together. When I ate meat, I started to realize that a dead animal was actually on my table. I just couldn't eat it anymore. I first stopped eating cows, then pigs, then chickens and turkeys. It was not until five years ago that I stopped eating dairy."

Advantages of being vegetarian: "I am always full of energy and have a large amount of stamina. Since strength and stamina play an important role, this is my advantage. I'm also able to play roles much younger than my age because of how healthy being vegan keeps me."

Challenges to being vegetarian: "Being on the road ten to eleven months of the year keeps me from eating my healthiest. I always make the best out of a situation with or without a fridge and kitchen."

Favorite preskate meal: pasta with tomato sauce, water, and sport drink

Favorite snacks: peanut butter and jelly sandwich, rice cakes, health-nut cookies

Favorite one-pot meal: Heath's Skating Mexican Fiesta Meal (page 95)

▼

PART TWO

Plant-Based Peak Performance

8

Supplementing the Sports Machine

s a world-class triathlete, six-time Hawaii Ironman champion, masters triathlete phenomenon, and 23-year vegetarian, Dave Scott recognizes the need to fuel the sports machine at 150% to race and function at peak performance levels. Dave, 44, is a triathlon camp director and coach to hundreds of Dave wanna-bes from the novice to the elite level.

Although Dave was macrobiotic for 2 years, he is currently a semivegetarian. Married and the father of three semivegetarians, Dave gave up meat when late work hours caused indigestion problems for meat-based dinners. He had other concerns about cholesterol and saturated fat, and environmental issues were mounting (see Preface).

Dave's current 1 1/2- to 3-hour training day doesn't warrant the same food intake as his 8-hour-per-day competitive training years. However, his middle-age maintenance program fueled him to a sixth-place finish in the 1996 Hawaiian Ironman at age 40 in 8 hours 38 minutes.

Dave drinks beer and/or wine once a week and takes no medications. He supplements his food intake with PowerBars three times daily, a multivitamin, vitamins E and C, beta-carotene, and iron. With this program, he claims to have "no ups or downs" in his training performance.

The 4-Billion-Dollar Question

Athletes at all levels of competition are searching for ways to gain a competitive advantage in their specific sport. According to triathlon legend Scott Tinley, "I'm not different. If the research looks credible, I'll swallow it."

—*Triathlon* magazine, September 1997

One of the first questions I am asked as a sports nutritionist and athlete is if I believe in supplements. My answer is yes and no.

First I work with an athlete's food intake, eating, and lifestyle behaviors to make sure the very best foods are being selected and consumed at appropriate times throughout the training period. I then massage the athlete's present lifestyle so that those most nutritious foods are purchased, stored, prepared, and consumed in comfortable and relaxing environments. Since athletes tend to eat on the run, foods are often not prepared safely in clean environments. Eating in transit forces the athlete to improperly chew food and eat excessive or deficient amounts.

All these factors will affect the bioavailability of nutrients from those foods and ruin the enjoyment of eating. After all, the peak performance diet is not just about getting potassium in a banana.

After I assess these factors, also discussed in chapter 7, I share my opinion about supplementation and the potential effects on sport performance. My answer is that some vitamin, mineral, and herbal supplements, including sport drinks, bars, and shakes, are extremely helpful and appropriate for certain groups of people at special times in training and life. However, supplements are not necessary for everyone all the time. In fact, for some, supplementation can do more harm than good . . . for health and for the pocket!

About 84% of world-class athletes take nutrient supplements, and 80% of the athletes profiled in this book use supplements for a variety of reasons. A list of their daily supplements is included on page 160.

> . . . when you're doing anything you can to gain a few seconds here or there, it's difficult to determine the effectiveness of one product over another. On the other hand, if you're dangerously

low in one particular mineral and happen to stumble upon a vehicle that will boost the levels, the newfound energy can be astounding.

—Scott Tinley, *Triathlon* magazine, September 1997

They're not alone. Supplements are used by at least 40 percent of all Americans. The Council for Responsible Nutrition has estimated the yearly retail dietary supplement expenditure as $4 billion per year, a number that increases each year.

In an effort to monitor dietary products more effectively and provide health-conscious consumers with better information about vitamins, herbs, and other dietary supplements, the Food and Drug Administration (FDA) require standardized "Supplement Facts" labels as of March 23, 1999.

The labels are similar to a food label, listing the product serving size, calories, and a complete list of ingredients. Well-established nutrients like vitamins A and C will appear at the top of the label with the "% Daily Value." A bar must separate other questionable ingredients.

Labels for herb products have additional requirements. The label must list the common name for the plant, the part of the plant used, and the amount in each tablet.

These government-imposed standards will help consumers use their money more wisely on supplement choices. These labels will also help athletes and others select products that will safely complement their present food choices. If in doubt, speak with a Registered Dietitian (RD) who specializes in plant-based diets for sports. A listing of groups that can refer you to a licensed and/or certified dietetic professional can be found in Appendix C.

In the meantime, this chapter will give you some information on the validity, safety, and consumption of supplements for sport performance. However, in no way are these supplement descriptions a recipe for your sports success.

In reality, the average vitamin and mineral intake of the VSNG athletes reflects no dietary deficiencies. Without supplements, their plant-based diets provide in excess of the RDA for most of the vitamins, minerals, and trace minerals. The athletes' dietary intakes that exceeded 100% of the RDAs are listed in the table on page 161.

▶ Top Supplement Choices of ◀
THE VEGETARIAN SPORTS NUTRITION GUIDE Athletes

Most popular supplements

Multivitamin (8)

Vitamin C (6)

Vitamin E (4)

Creatine (4)

None (3)

Iron (2)

Protein powders or drinks (2)

Beta-carotene (2)

PowerBars (2)

Supplements primarily taken by one athlete*

Vitamin B$_{12}$

Calcium

Green Foods: super blue
green, algae, spirulina,
and/or chlorella

Mix: yeast, lecithin,
wheat germ, and
molasses oat bran

Bee pollen

Plant-based colloidal minerals

Enzymes

E-Mergen-C

Vitamin B complex

Sport drinks

Nutri Rx with creatine

Chromium

St. John's wort

Echinachea

Goldenseal

Glucosamine and sodium
chondroitin

Drinks—green tea/caffeine

Arginine drink

Ginkgo biloba

Pycnogenol

Grapeseed

Phosphatidylserine

Melatonin

Magnesium malate

Alphalipoic acid

Whey protein

Carnitine

Glucosamine

Glutamine

Glutathione

Panax Ginseng

Note: The number in parentheses indicates how many of the 17 athletes use this supplement.

* Most of the supplements on the "single" supplement list are consumed on a regular basis by double ironman champion Gary Gromet. Maybe he knows something we do not, or he is just fortunate to own a health food and supplement store and have these products readily available to him. (See page 238 for Gary's profile.)

► VSNG Spotlight Athletes' Dietary Intakes of Vitamins ◄ and Minerals* that Exceeded 100% of the RDAs

VITAMIN OR MINERAL	AMOUNT CONSUMED	RDA	% RDA
Vitamin A	3,000 RE (9,990 IU)	1,000 (RE)	300
Thiamin, B$_1$ (mg)	2.9	1.2	239
Riboflavin, B$_2$ (mg)	2.2	1.4	160
Niacin, B$_3$ (mg)	29.0	15	192
Pyridoxine, B$_6$	3.3	2	163
Folate (μg)	656.0	200	328
Vitamin B$_{12}$ (μg)	3.7	2	184
Vitamin C (mg)	327.0	60	546
Vitamin K (μg)	421.0	80	526
Potassium (mg)	4,374.0	2,000	219
Phosphorus (mg)	1,736.0	800	217
Magnesium (mg)	569.0	350	163
Iron (mg)	22.0	10	217
Manganese (mg)	7.7	3.5	220
Selenium (mg)	0.15	.070	214
Copper (mg)	2.4	1.5–3	105

(RE): Retinol Equivalents

(μg): Micrograms

*Average dietary intakes (excluding supplements) of 12–15 athletes, excluding myself.

These VSNG athletes received substantial but not overadequate RDAs of biotin, 50%; vitamin D, 54%; vitamin E, 82%; sodium, 66%; zinc, 72%; and calcium, 95%.

For vegan athletes Ben, Ruth, Charlene, and Craig, an average of their daily consumption of vitamins and minerals through food showed levels of 79% to 538% of the RDAs for all nutrients except biotin and vitamin D.

It's obvious that a plant-based diet will provide adequate amounts of vitamins and minerals. But do athletes training and competing at a higher level need more? Do recreational athletes have special needs?

Remember some of the questions you asked yourself in chapter 7 regarding the impact of your health status, training intensity, environmental training conditions, food purchasing habits, and other factors that may affect your vitamin and mineral status. What does the research have to say about supplementation and sports perform-ance?

Research Says . . .

Most reliable research does not justify the need for extra single or combination vitamin supplements except when the athlete is in a defi-ciency state. Too often, insufficient data, limited subjects and controls, no diet relationship, or a sport-specific discipline investigated under uncontrolled conditions is used to look at the value and benefits of a vitamin, mineral, or other compound for performance.

This leaves sports nutritionists (RD) more limited in the advice they offer on supplementation. However, it does not deter the individuals selling, promoting, or testifying on behalf of the miracle values of any supplement. Therefore, the athlete is vulnerable to advertisements touting the benefits of a specific supplement on speed, energy, and/or endurance. To the competitive or professional athlete, this can be very tempting; better performance times mean money back in his or her pocket. Promoting others' products regardless of results in exchange for sponsorship funding can be a significant source of income for the sub-world-class athlete and others.

This cutting-edge review summarizes some of the most popular supplements and/or other substances consumed by athletes, along with the best research available at the time of finishing this book. Keep in mind that this research seems to be updated weekly.

The B Vitamins

The B vitamins are involved in energy production from carbohydrates and fats and with red blood cell formation. The rationale for using sup-plements is due to their physiological effect on the athlete and the fact that prolonged deficiency can affect endurance performance. Since cooking and the use of certain medications can affect nutrient absorption, it may be likely that a secondary deficiency exists. Signs of potential deficiencies are described in chapter 7. Therefore, it seems logical that any activity requiring additional energy would jus-tify the need for extra B's.

Thiamin—B_1

Various reports suggest a definitive link between high carbohydrate intakes, physical exertion, and thiamin needs. Vigorous exercise is accompanied by an increased demand for thiamin for energy and protein breakdown, specifically the Branched chain amino acids (BCAAs). Moderate exercise is not reported to have this same effect. Although many reports on thiamin and exercise do not include detailed dietary information, several researchers suggest that thiamin intakes in the range of two to three times the RDA of 1.5–3 milligrams/day is adequate for the increased energy demands of moderate aerobic exercise. Only those on high-carbohydrate diets would benefit from a higher daily dose. Further studies are needed, however.

Riboflavin—B_2

Although riboflavin supplementation has not been shown to enhance performance, riboflavin (B_2) is involved in protecting hemoglobin, and hemoglobin carries oxygen to muscles. In B_2-deficient athletes, riboflavin needs may increase; however, supplementation for the adequately fed athlete is not warranted.

Niacin—B_3

Niacin (B_3) also delivers oxygen to the working muscle. Niacin helps with fat, carbohydrate, hormone, and tissue metabolism. It is speculated that taking large doses of niacin can actually be detrimental to performance by causing an increase in glycogen use and a decrease in blood fats and fats used from adipose during exercise. In addition, if more glycogen is used, more lactic acid is produced, inhibiting fat as an energy source. Therefore, based on current evidence, there is no need or advantage for niacin supplementation in sport.

Pyridoxine—B_6

Pyridoxine (B_6) is needed for protein metabolism. A deficiency decreases glycogen used for energy and hemoglobin formation. High-protein diets may warrant higher needs; however, research with athletes does not justify the need for supplements, nor does it show enhanced effects on sports performance with additional doses of pyridoxine. Since a toxicity can cause paralysis and other nerve-related conditions, supplementation is not advised.

Folate and Cobalamin—B_{12}

Folic acid (folate in food) is involved in DNA production and red blood cell formation. Vitamin B_{12} protects nerve fibers and works hand in hand with folate to manufacture red blood cells. A deficiency in B_{12}, folate, or B_6 can cause a type of anemia called "pernicious anemia." Since B_{12} is found primarily in animal products, vegans need to consume fortified foods, sport bars, shakes, and/or supplements that meet daily needs.

Despite this potential concern, athletes from controlled studies have not been found to be deficient in these B vitamins. Supplements and injections of B_{12} have been used by athletes to improve energy levels, but there is no evidence to support this practice in non-deficient individuals.

Other B vitamin deficiency concerns brought to the public's attention are the relationship between these vitamins and heart disease. A deficiency of B_{12}, B_6, or folate can lead to coronary problems. Folate deficiency anemia can affect the fetuses of pregnant women; therefore, folic acid has recently been added to the fortification list on processed foods.

Pantothenic Acid and Biotin

Pantothenic acid and biotin regulate many metabolic processes that are important for exercise performance. Pantothenic acid is a part of acetyl CoA, involved in the manufacturing and use of fatty acids and pyruvate. Biotin is also part of the complex pyruvate needs to make glucose for energy. Deficiencies have not been reported with pantothenic acid. Because intestinal microorganisms can synthesize biotin, deficiencies are also rarely seen in this B vitamin. Minimal research has been devoted to the effects of supplementation on performance, yet athletes generally take these vitamins as a part of a B-complex formula. Supplementation is not warranted at this time.

Vitamin C

Vitamin C is the most popular supplement of this book's athletes and the most popular supplement used by the public. Vitamin C plays a critical role in many functions important to sports performance, as described in chapter 7. Research shows that a slight deficiency can affect performance and immunity in the athlete.

Research also shows that levels of vitamin C can fall after long-distance running. In one study, runners who consumed 600 milligrams of vitamin C three weeks before a 42K race developed fewer upper respiratory infections than unsupplemented runners. Another study showed less muscle soreness in athletes who consumed 3 grams of vitamin C before and 4 grams after strenuous calf muscle exercises.

Since the amount of vitamin C is further reduced by cooking or by the consumption of certain medications, exercising in the heat, smog, cigarette smoke, and heavy metal exposure and large amounts may be lost in sweat, supplementation may be reasonable in a suggested range of 100–500 mg per day. Some things you need to consider before you run out for your next bottle of vitamin C are:

▶ Although supplements may be warranted, there are few studies in which vitamin C has been used as a sole antioxidant before an exercise bout.

▶ Chronic multiple doses can increase kidney stones, decrease blood coagulation time, and cause GI problems. Long-term use can even cause iron-overload cardiac death (caused by the ability of C to improve iron absorption).

My recommendations for supplementing with the water-soluble vitamins are:

Vegetarian athletes can meet their vitamin B and vitamin C needs through healthy grain, bean, pea, vegetable, and fruit choices. None of the spotlight athletes' diets were deficient in these vitamins, with the exception of biotin. However, this vitamin can be replenished internally.

If one wants to supplement the water-soluble vitamins and maintain energy levels while doing so, it is best to get the vitamins by eating a sport bar daily. Some of the sport bars, such as PowerBar Harvest, Forza Bullet, GeniSoy Protein Bar, Balance, and Gary Null's Bar, all provide a minimum of 20 to 50% of the RDAs for the B vitamins. PowerBar, Stoker, Ultrafuel, and Tiger Sport provide 100%. All bars provide 100% of vitamin C. Ultrafuel provides 420%.

Another avenue of supplementation is fluid supplements. Two products on the market are Greens Today, by The Organic Frog Company, and E-Mergen-C, by Alacer. These supplements are easy to use.

They come in individualized packets of powder, which are easy to take on the road and blend with water or juice.

I enjoy blending Greens Today, a soy-based protein formula made with 23 grams of soy isoflavones, 72 other phytochemicals, vitamins, and minerals, with ice and water after some of my morning workouts. It is plentiful in vitamins B and C. It also has about 176 calories of carbohydrates and protein energy.

E-Mergen-C is an effervescent, calorie-free supplement that Chris Campbell and I both use. When added to water, this "fizz" drink provides an abundance of B vitamins, 1,000 milligrams of vitamin C, and the electrolytes. Since I'm a heavy sweater and real vitamin/mineral loser, this is my favorite supplement during long, hot, humid Miami runs and ironman distance events during the summer months. They have a variety of flavors; however, I enjoy the cranberry flavor. See the additional benefits of cranberries on vegetarian diets in chapter 6.

Fat-Soluble Vitamins

Few studies suggest the need for additional amounts of fat-soluble vitamins or their positive influence on physical performance. While vitamins D and K and beta-carotene supplements have not been shown to improve performance, and in fact can be toxic in supplemental form, athletes should focus on consuming foods rich in these vitamins. Recent evidence has suggested a potential link between beta-carotene supplementation and an increased risk of lung cancer. Since vegetarian athletes have no problem consuming enough greens and orange-colored vegetables or getting enough sunlight or fortified milk and dairy substitutes to meet their daily needs, supplementing with vitamins A, D, and K is not warranted.

Supplementing with vitamin E may have some validity under special conditions. Although vitamin E deficiencies are rare, athletes who maintain a high-carbohydrate, low-fat diet may have a low intake. There is also some evidence to suggest that supplemental vitamin E as an antioxidant may augment oxidative muscle stress, especially in untrained individuals and the elderly. At altitude, vitamin E supplements showed improvements in VO2max, decreased submaximal oxygen intake, and reduced oxygen debt. It has not, however, been shown to have a performance-enhancing effect in elite athletes training at sea level. Therefore, a need for supplementation can be satisfied by consuming fortified sport bars, cereals, and sport drinks like Perform by PowerBar. You can also get extra vitamin E by sprinkling wheat germ on your favorite vegetable dish.

Minerals

Iron

Athletes who may be at increased risk for iron deficiency, such as regular and heavily menstruating females, endurance athletes, and low-body-weight and long-distance runners, may benefit from iron supplementation. The total iron losses may be as high as 2 milligrams per day in runners from sweat and GI bleeding.

The vegetarian athletes in this book consume adequate amounts of iron through their dietary choices. Sport bars, shakes, and supplements provide additional amounts.

Therefore, unless an athlete has been diagnosed as having iron deficiency anemia, too much dietary iron inhibits zinc absorption, stimulates "free radicals," and may lead to heart disease. Male athletes should not take supplements unless a deficiency has been diagnosed. For others, 18 to 50 milligrams of ferrous sulfate appears to be the most effective in raising the athlete's serum ferritin levels.

To improve the intake and availability of iron without supplementation:

▶ Do not consume calcium and iron products together at the same meal.

▶ Limit the amount of fiber with high-iron meals.

▶ Take a citrus source of at least 100 milligrams of vitamin C with an iron-rich food to increase absorption up to 400%.

The Electrolytes

Potassium

Getting enough potassium is not usually a problem for vegetarian athletes and other plant-based eaters. Supplements are generally not recommended except under extreme conditions such as sweating and diarrhea. Under other conditions, potassium losses are negligible.

Potassium supplements can actually be potentially dangerous. Abnormally high levels of potassium in the blood can result in cardiac arrhythmia.

Sodium and Chloride

Deficiencies in these minerals from excessive sweating, critical for the maintenance of fluids and nerve impulses for muscle contraction, are not desirable. If you've had the chance to see or participate in a long, hot marathon or ironman competition, then you know about the IV line at the end of the race. Replacements of the electrolytes are key to success and life!

Since consuming an excess of water during endurance exercise may also result in hyponatremia (low sodium in the blood) and cause drowsiness, muscle weakness, cramping, confusion, and seizures, sport drinks with electrolytes are recommended for the long haul.

Author's suggestion: Consume sport drinks like Gatorade on a hot day, and snack on salted low-fat chips and other salty snacks. These drinks and foods can actually be beneficial to the tropically trained or racing athlete. Since vegetarians are known to limit their intake of processed foods, their diets are often found to be lower in sodium than others. Salting some of your favorite dishes and seasoning some of the VSNG recipes is recommended and desirable.

Zinc

In relation to performance, zinc has several functions that may be important. Since zinc regulates the activity of enzymes linked to energy metabolism in the cell, zinc may be lost during strenuous exercise. Exercise has been shown to increase zinc loss from the body. One of the drawbacks to long-term supplementation is the lowering of high-density lipoprotein (HDL) cholesterol (see chapter 5), protective against heart disease.

Author's suggestion: Zinc is easy to find in fortified sport bars, cereals, and shakes. To maximize zinc absorption, try the following:

Drink tea and coffee between meals.

Emphasize the high-zinc VSNG recipes and snacks in your peak performance diet.

Use zinc-fortified foods as needed.

Calcium

Since calcium is necessary for muscle contraction and other life and structural functions, it is always demanded. Although not a problem nutrient in vegetarian athletes, in amenorrheic or postmenopausal women low calcium intakes and low estrogen levels may require additional calcium to reach a level of 1,500 mg day to achieve balance. Even though there are no ergogenic effects associated with calcium supplementation, an adequate amount is suggested to maintain performance.

Author's suggestion: Sport bars and shakes, fortified soy milks, and low-fat dairy are good sources of calcium. Recently, foods in the general market such as cottage cheese, orange juice, tofu, yogurt, soy milk, and other dairy alternatives have been fortified with calcium. Even gum and water have included calcium in their formulas!

Selenium

Selenium functions with vitamin E to protect cells from damage. Little research on its effects on sports performance exists, except in conjunction with other antioxidant supplements. Selenium supplements could be extremely toxic. Using Charlene's Skating Supplement, sprinkling wheat germ on your morning cereal or on Stephen's No Horsing Around Vegetable Plate (chapter 7, page 150), or having your morning oats with bran and orange juice can provide a selenium-rich, plant-based way to start your day.

Charlene's Skating Supplement

Makes 1 serving

1 tsp wheat germ

1 tsp molasses

1 tsp oat bran

$1/4$ oz lecithin

1 tsp brewer's yeast

▶ Nutrients per serving: 86 calories, 2 grams protein, 8 grams carbohydrate, 7 grams fat, 3 grams sugar

▶ Dietary composition: 8% protein, 31% carbohydrates, 61% fat

▶ VSNG food servings: ½ grain, 1 fat

▶ Good source of folate; moderate source of vitamin B_1 and phosphorus

Charlene adds her supplement to juice or oatmeal and takes it a couple of times per week.

Charlene's Skating Supplement added to ½ cup orange juice

▶ Nutrients per serving: 142 calories, 3 grams protein, 21 grams carbohydrates, 7 grams fat

▶ Dietary composition: 7% protein, 53% carbohydrates, 40% fat

▶ VSNG food servings: 1 fruit, 1 fat

▶ Good source of vitamin B_1, C, folate, phosphorus

Charlene's Skating Supplement added to oatmeal

▶ Nutrients per serving: 231 calories, 8 grams protein, 33 grams carbohydrates, 9 grams fat, 2 grams saturated fat, 1 gram monounsaturated fat, 1 gram linoleic fat, 4 grams sugar, 3 grams fiber

▶ Dietary composition: 13% protein, 54% carbohydrates, 33% fat

▶ VSNG food servings: 2 grains, 1 fat

▶ Good source of vitamin B_1, folate, phosphorus, manganese; moderate source of vitamin E, magnesium, selenium

---

Copper

Copper is associated with oxygen transport. A deficiency can potentially cause energy problems in the athlete. Since copper in supplement form acts like an emetic (causes vomiting), singular supplements are not advised. A high intake of zinc, vitamin C, iron, and other minerals may decrease the absorption. Therefore, the best supplemental sources are sport bars, shakes, nuts, and legumes. Erika's Trail Mix prepared with Brazil nuts, almonds, hazelnuts, or walnuts can also provide an additional dietary source.

Phosphorus

Phosphate loading has been shown to increase anaerobic threshold and improve buffering capacity and cardiovascular response to exercise. This refers to the ingestion of a large amount of phosphate in the form of a salt, 4 grams per day for several days before a competitive event. High doses act like a drug by elevating red blood cells, increasing oxygen delivery to tissues, and enhancing performance.

Studies support a 1-gram, neutral-buffered sodium phosphate four times per day for three days prior to competition. In male long-distance runners, this dose has been associated with an increase in maximum oxygen consumption (VO2max) and an increase in blood lactate. A six-day loading period has been shown to increase hemoglobin levels in another group of runners.

Author's recommendation: Do not take phosphate salts for extended periods of time, since they can interfere with calcium levels. Phos Fuel, a supplement by Twinlab, has the dose recommended to achieve the desired goal of phosphate loading in an easy-to-take pill. In addition, B vitamins including biotin are included in the supplement.

Magnesium

Magnesium's primary function is enzyme activation. Several studies have shown that after exercise, magnesium is lost from the body. While sweat is responsible for a small part of the loss, urine is the main culprit. In one study of marathon runners, magnesium losses increased until 12 hours after the race. It was speculated that pH changes or hormone changes were responsible.

Author's suggestion: Athletes who train heavily on a daily basis might need additional magnesium. Although sport bars such as Power-Bar and Stoker provide some additional magnesium, E-Mergen-C supplement is also an option for endurance training on long, hot days. You can also try Ruth's Ironwoman Pho (Vietnamese soup) in chapter 7 (page 149), rich in this and other essential vitamins and minerals. Other great supplemental sources include Charlene's Skating Supplement (pages 169–170), trail mix with almonds or cashews, or a tofu and buckwheat dish sprinkled with wheat germ, soybeans, corn, and peas.

Don't Lose the Vitamins and Minerals

Vitamin losses occur with the passage of time from modern agricultural methods that produce vitamin-deficient crops, transportation, storage, refining, further processing, and cooking. Exposure to oxygen (called oxidation), light, or heat, changes in acidity (pH), and the physical separation of vitamins from food are responsible. Some of the vitamin losses due to handling are described in the table below.

▶ Vitamin and Mineral Losses in Food ◀

VITAMIN/MINERAL	CAUSE OF LOSSES
A and D	light, air, and acid; stable in cooking
E	light, air, and high-temperature frying; unstable in fried foods during frozen storage
K	low or high acid conditions and light
C	one of the most easily destroyed vitamins; exposure to light or heat; contact with iron or copper utensils; minimal destruction when fruits and vegetables are placed immediately in boiling water, maximal if placed in cold water and slowly brought to the boil (use little water, place lid on saucepan immediately to exclude air, and serve immediately); dehydration in making instant potato granules destroys most of the vitamin C
Pyridoxine (B_6)	heat and light
Biotin	heat
Pantothenic acid and folate	heat, air, light, and acid; 50% folate is lost in canning and after cooking vegetables
B_{12}	pasteurization of milk destroys 7%; boiling for 3 minutes destroys 30%
Thiamin (B_1) and riboflavin (B_2)	heat, air, and low-acid environments; 40% lost when canned food liquids are discarded; 50% B_2 lost from milk in 2 hours by exposure to bright sunlight
Calcium, iron, phosphorus, magnesium	boiling, minerals leached into surrounding water and juice
Potassium and sodium	minerals lost in discarded canned juice

The best way to prevent nutrient losses is by purchasing foods locally grown and sold at farmer's markets and co-ops. Choose fresh, unprocessed fruits, grains, and whole grains, or enriched and/or fortified foods if fresh is unavailable. Store the foods away from light and heat and prepare them with minimal temperature, water, and handling. Microwaving has actually been shown to prevent excessive losses of vitamin C and folic acid when compared with traditional methods of preparation, so athletes on the run need not worry about using the hotel substitute cooking facilities.

Vitamin Interference

Taking medications, eating certain foods, or drinking caffeine or alcohol can interfere with the absorption or metabolism of vitamins and minerals. These dietary nuisances can make nutrients unavailable for absorption, alter food intake by modifying taste and appetite, and/or interfere with vitamin and mineral absorption from food.

Prescription, over-the-counter (OTC), and illegal medicines can do harm because they interfere with the body's normal use of nutrients. Some compounds naturally occurring in food, such as fiber, phytates, tannins, and oxalates, can also bind important minerals in foods. Legal medications that can interfere with absorption include oral contraceptives, antibiotics, aspirin, caffeine, diuretics, laxatives, and estrogen replacement therapy. Illegal drugs such as amphetamines, steroids, cocaine, and marijuana can also radically increase or decrease an individual's appetite and consequently effect vitamin and mineral status.

Some of the effects of drinks and drugs on nutrient absorption are described in the Drug–Nutrient Interactions table on page 174.

Other Popular Supplements

Chromium

According to the National Research Council of the American Academy of Sciences, 50 to 90% of Americans fail to take in the daily requirement of chromium. Situations such as stress, high sugar intake, diabetes, physical trauma and infections, and strenuous exercise, as well as food processing, are all associated with compromised chromium status.

▶ Drug–Nutrient Interactions ◀

DRUG	EFFECT ON ABSORPTION, EXCRETION, OR METABOLISM
Legal	
Alcohol	potential deficiencies in B_1, B_3, pantothenic acid, folate, vitamin C, magnesium, phosphorus
Antibiotics	reduce fat, amino acid, folate, fat-soluble vitamins, B_{12}, copper, iron, magnesium, potassium, phosphate, and zinc absorption; interfere with vitamin K synthesis
Anti-depressants	increase or curb appetite; increase cravings for simple carbohydrates
Aspirin	lowers folate; increase excretion of B_1, vitamin C, vitamin K, iron, potassium
Caffeine	increases excretion of calcium and magnesium; may elevate blood cholesterol
Diuretics	interfere with zinc storage; lower blood folate, chloride, magnesium, phosphorus, potassium, B_{12}, calcium, sodium, B_1
Estrogen replacement therapy	reduces folate, causes sodium absorption; may raise blood sugar and triglycerides and lower vitamin C, B_6, B_2, calcium, magnesium, zinc
Laxatives	reduce absorption of glucose, fat, beta-carotene, vitamin D, E, and K, calcium, phosphate, potassium
Oral contraceptives	reduce folate, B_2, B_6, B_{12}, vitamin C absorption; cause sodium retention; possibly improve absorption of calcium; low levels of serum (blood) zinc and iron in some women
Illegal	
Marijuana	alters taste and appetite; enhanced enjoyment of sweets; reduced nutrient density of diet due to high-calorie, low-quality foods
Cocaine	reduces appetite; consequences of starvation—loss of muscle mass, weight, water, nutrients; may lead to eating disorders
Food Compounds	
Avidin	egg white protein that binds biotin when uncooked
Oxalates	organic acids found in spinach, rhubarb, beet greens, and chocolate; interfere with calcium and iron absorption
Phytates	found in the husks of grains, legumes, seeds; bind calcium, magnesium, zinc, iron
Tannins	found in tea and some grains; interfere with iron absorption

Since chromium helps insulin regulate blood sugar, a deficiency may cause glucose intolerance. Chromium is found primarily in plant-based foods such as asparagus, mushrooms, prunes, nuts, whole-grain breads, cereals, brewer's yeast, and beer. Since chromium has a low absorption rate, supplement manufacturers have bound it to piccolate to increase bioavailability.

Chromium supplementation became popular when press reports highlighted its reported enhancement of fat, protein, and carbohydrate metabolism and body fat losses. In the 1980s, researchers demonstrated an anabolic steroid effect with dosages of 200 µg/day. None of these studies has been reproduced.

Although no side effects have been associated with doses of 50–200 µg/day for less than one month, other reports show that the picolinic acid in chromium piccolate supplements may cause anemia, cognitive (mind) impairment, and kidney problems. Caution should be exercised.

Alkaline Salts

One of the potential mechanisms of muscular fatigue is the accumulation of hydrogen in the system, which causes a drop in the blood's pH, inhibits the release of calcium to help muscles contract, reduces the activity of glycolytic enzymes hat use sugars for energy, and impairs neural impulses. As exercise progresses, the blood and muscle's natural buffering systems, including bicarbonate, try to "capture" hydrogen and delay a drop in muscular pH. Theoretically, the ingestion of additional alkaline salts could build the body's buffering capacity and therefore delay the onset of fatigue.

Over 30 human investigations have examined the potential ergogenic effect of sodium bicarbonate as a supplement. The findings have been very inconsistent and contradictory. However, supplementation with sodium bicarbonate may be effective in high-intensity exercise lasting 1 to 10 minutes or high-intensity exercise with intermittent, short rest periods.

Author's suggestion: The available evidence suggests a loading dose of 0.3 grams sodium bicarbonate per kilogram body weight (along with a liter of water) to enhance high-intensity exercise performance. However, take caution because some athletes may experience abdominal

pain, bloating, nausea, or "explosive" diarrhea one hour after ingestion. Long-term use may cause muscle spasms, gastric rupture, or cardiac arrhythmia.

Beta-Hydroxy-Beta-Methylbutyrate

Beta-hydroxy-beta-methylbutyrate (HMB) is a metabolite of the amino
acid leucine (one of the branched chain amino acids, or BCAAs).
About 5 to 10% of leucine is converted to HMB. In muscle and white
blood cells, HMB may be important for cholesterol synthesis, muscle
cell integrity, and function.

A dose-related effect has been shown from taking up to 3 grams
per day. The current recommended dosage of 1.5 to 3 grams of HMB
per day was given to forty male volunteers who participated in a resis-
tance-training program. The results showed that HMB supplements
were associated with greater increase in muscle mass and strength
when compared with a placebo. In exercising women, HMB supplementation resulted in increased lean muscle gain and strength.

In endurance training, HMB supplements may slow the effects of
delayed-onset muscle soreness caused by muscle damage. In a recent
study with runners, significant decreases in muscle damage were
shown.

HMB has been shown to have a wide margin of safety. In addition,
a 6 to 12% reduction of blood cholesterol has been demonstrated with
supplementation. Three grams per day combined with resistance
training and/or endurance training appears to be beneficial.

Creatine

Creatine is an amino acid synthesized in the body from the amino
acids glycine, methionine, and arginine at a rate of 1 gram per day. Creatine also comes from meat in the diet. However, the amount in meat
drops significantly after cooking.

Studies show that 20 to 30 grams of creatine supplements may
increase the storage of creatine and creatine phosphate (CP) for short-
term anaerobic exercise. CP also buffers excess hydrogen associated
with lactate production and fatigue. Like glycogen loading, discussed
in chapter 4, or phosphate loading, discussed in this chapter, creatine
dosages need to be loaded for maximum benefits. Unlike carbohydrate

loading, creatine loading is most effective in preseason training to help enhance training and performance.

Research suggests that an initial phase of four to five 5-gram doses every three to four waking hours for five to six days will keep blood levels of creatine elevated throughout the day and increase the uptake of creatine to skeletal muscle. Since its uptake is enhanced by insulin, each dose should be taken with food.

After this loading phase, a daily maintenance dose of 5 grams per day is adequate to compensate for the normal daily turnover of creatine (about 2 grams per day) and to maintain elevated creatine levels in muscle. Amounts greater than 5 grams are excreted in urine.

Although there are no serious side effects to supplementation with these doses, a slight gain in body weight has been reported and may compromise short-distance racing performance.

L-Carnitine

Carnitine transports fat across the cell membrane, where it is used for energy. It is synthesized in the liver and kidneys from the amino acids lysine and methionine, and found in meats and dairy products. Therefore, vegetarians might need supplements.

Carnitine may provide a more efficient use of energy. It may be ergogenic and prolong exercise by sparing glycogen and by buffering pyruvate. Since it moves fat across the cell membrane, increased availability from supplements may facilitate more use of fats. Long-term research of eight weeks and longer has shown promising results. Other research has had equivocal results. The jury's still out!

Coenzyme Q10 (CoQ10)

As a vitamin-like substance, CoQ10 plays a role as an antioxidant and free radical scavenger. Studies show that CoQ10 tissue levels peak at age 20, then decline. The amount in the hearts of heart disease patients is lower. In fact, many studies show that CoQ10 can alleviate symptoms of heart disease.

Despite positive results with rats, humans have not demonstrated the same effects with supplementation. Based on current research, the benefits for athletes are speculative at best. However, no toxic effects have been reported with 100 mg of CoQ10, outside of GI distress.

Pyruvate

Pyruvate is produced at the end stages of glucose breakdown. Improved endurance with supplementation is supported by two studies, one of which evaluated supplementation on arm endurance and another on leg endurance. In the first study, 25 grams of pyruvate taken with 75 grams of dihydroxyacetone (DHA) was shown to increase arm muscle glucose extraction and enhance endurance. In the second study, the results were duplicated in conjunction with a high-carbohydrate diet. However, other studies have not reproduced these results, and show the benefits of DHA/pyruvate supplements on weight loss in two trials.

Below are listed potential concerns regarding these studies.

▶ Since the subjects were untrained, it is questionable whether supplements would work with elite or trained athletes.

▶ Possible gas, flatus, and diarrhea are side effects.

▶ Commercial preparations contain more pyruvate (500 mg–1 gram) and may not contain DHA. There is no guarantee of consistent dosage.

Glycerol

Glycerol, also called glycerine, is a natural component of many foods and is also added to processed foods. Recent research suggests that when a glycerol and water mix is used as a hydration beverage, performance may be improved. Glycerol does this by making better use of water by encouraging the body to act like a sponge. After ingestion, it is rapidly absorbed and distributed throughout the body, holding onto water and delaying dehydration.

In one cycling study, athletes were able to pedal 29% longer with lower heart rates and temperatures when compared with water-only exercise bouts. Important considerations include using food-grade glycerol and limiting the dose to 1 gram per kilogram of body weight every 6 hours. Exceeding this dosage can cause bloating, nausea, and lightheadedness.

Dehydroepiandrosterone

Dehydroepiandrosterone (DHEA), an androgen produced in the adrenal glands, was pulled from the market in 1996 by the FDA until its safety had been reviewed. It is a precursor of androgens and estrogens and is found in wild yams. DHEA may increase the production of testosterone and provide an anabolic steroid effect. Claims range from slowing the aging process to psychological well-being. Its effect on healthy individuals younger than 40 years old is unstudied.

To competitive athletes, a positive testosterone–epitesterone ratio exceeding 6:1 can be a result (remember Mary Decker Slaney's past problems?). Therefore, professional athletes should stay away from this one!

It has also been shown to have other undesirable effects, including irreversible virilization in women, hair loss, voice deepening in females, and irreversible gynecomastia from elevated estrogen levels in men. Supplementation is not recommended.

Androstenedione

Banned by the IOC and most health organizations, androstenedione, pronounced "andro-STEEN-die-own," is an androgenic anabolic steroid (AAS) and only differs from testosterone by a hydrogen atom. It's produced by the adrenal glands, ovaries, and testes and is a precursor to testosterone and estrogen.

Although its effect is dependent on many factors, including hormone control, enzymes, and digestion, it's probably not used, metabolized, and then excreted by the body. However, the effects could be similar to steroid use, including abnormal menstrual cycles, acne, excessive facial hair, liver dysfunction, increased LDL and decreased HDL cholesterol (see chapter 5), enlargement of the clitoris (may be permanent), and heart problems for women. For men, you can add kidney disease, shrunken testicles, premature baldness, and "roid rage."

Research on the short- and long-term effects using well-designed studies has not been conducted. The short- and long-term effects are inconclusive; therefore, athletes need to stay away from this one!

Vanadium (Vanadyl Sulfate)

Vanadium is a trace mineral (see chapter 7), although its essentiality is not clear. The normal diet provides about 12 to 28 mcg per day. Although increased muscle mass, vascularity, glycogen synthesis and storage, and anabolic effects are some of the claims, supplements have caused abdominal pain, anorexia, and weight loss. More serious side effects on glutathione, vitamin C, fats, and developmental toxicities have been shown in animal research. This is not recommended as a dietary supplement.

Herbs

Some athletes consume herbs in tablets, teas, and capsules to enhance performance. They feel that because the Chinese have proven their effectiveness over the last 2,000 years, and because they are more natural than vitamins, they are safe.

Many of the popular herbs have been reviewed in chapter 6 in the lifestyle beverages section. Ma huang warrants additional discussion.

Ma huang (ephedra)

Similar in structure to amphetamines, ma huang, better known as ephedra, increases heart rate and blood pressure. According to the FDA, 8 people have died and 500 made ill by dietary supplements containing ephedra. It is considered illegal by the International Olympic Committee (IOC) and the National Collegiate Athletic Association (NCAA).

The FDA has also described serious adverse effects associated with chaparral, comfrey, lobelia, germander, willow bark yohimbe, and Chinese herbal preparations containing stephania and magnolia. In addition, allergic reactions to bee pollen and others can occur in susceptible individuals. The best reference for herbal information is by Varro Tyler, Ph.D., and is listed in chapter 6 and in Appendix C.

To Supplement or Not to Supplement?

After reading this chapter, you may just feel like you need extra vitamins and minerals to excel at your favorite sport. Perhaps it hasn't affected your decision to take a supplement. Maybe you feel so good on your present supplement program, regardless of the information presented here, that you'd rather not mess with a good thing.

If you choose to take a supplement, there are some guidelines you can follow to ensure you have the best formula for peak performance training and competition.

▶ Consult with a sports nutritionist (RD) to evaluate your need for a supplement and the best dosage. It pays to have your diet evaluated first prior to consuming an arbitrary amount that may actually do more harm than good.

▶ Compare your present supplements with the Recommended Dietary Allowances for age and gender. Rule of thumb is to purchase one that has 100% of your RDA or very close to that amount. "High-potency" and therapeutic doses just mean more, and more is not always better.

▶ Avoid any preparation that has 10 times the RDA of vitamin A, D, or any mineral. Not only can these vitamins be toxic at high doses, but minerals can interact with others and fail to be absorbed. For example, zinc binds copper and calcium, iron hinders zinc, calcium hinders magnesium and iron, and magnesium binds calcium and iron. Even certain herbs can interfere with the absorption of nutrients and foods, so use caution.

▶ Avoid taking high amounts of iron. More than 10 milligrams per day is unnecessary except for those athletes deficient in iron. Too much can increase the risk for heart disease.

▶ Avoid organic or natural preparations (just in this case, not in food). They are no better than the standard preparations and cost much more. Synthetic may sound fake, but it just means put together. Synthetic vitamins are the same as the other expensive types.

▶ Stress formulas are blends of the B vitamins and C. There is no evidence to show that this will actually help you overcome stress. Try a run, warm shower, and massage. It's cheaper than a supply of these pills.

▶ Colloidal mixtures, the hottest supplements to arrive on the scene, are no more than minerals suspended in liquid clay. When water is mixed with clay, the elements are released. Manufacturers claim that colloidal suspensions supply trace minerals with uniquely high bioavailability. Since the mixture relies on the quantities in the clay, the amounts you see on the bottle are not always what you get. Research has shown anywhere from undetectable levels of minerals to excessive and toxic amounts of aluminum, lead, and strontium. The final word is that colloidals may be toxic and unsafe and would be a major waste of money.

▶ Liquid versus solid pills: More often than not, both are absorbed equally well. It's a matter of personal preference.

▶ Time-released formulations are intended to prevent the rapid and abrupt rise in the blood stream by dissolving slowly in the intestine. However, your body does not recognize the difference. Time-released or not, vitamins and minerals are absorbed at very specific sites along the intestine. Once they move past the absorption site, it is less likely that they will be absorbed later. Therefore nutrients from time-released preparations may be poorly absorbed.

On a final note, save your money and spend it on some new and exciting plant-based food choices, sport bars, and shakes. These foods and beverages will give you extra vitamins and minerals as well as energy. Turn to chapters 9 and 10 to learn the best way to eat with *The Vegetarian Sports Nutrition Guide* peak performance guide to eating.

Spotlight Athlete

Dave Scott

Professional triathlete, six-time Hawaiian Ironman World Champion

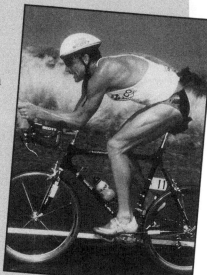

Age: 43

22 years vegetarian (macrobiotic 2 years); currently semivegetarian

Reason for becoming vegetarian: "Environmental concern of beef industry affecting resources, water, pollution, land availability. Secondly, I was working late and beef did not settle well. Third, I reduced cholesterol and saturated fat."

Advantages of being vegetarian: "No ups or downs with training/performance. Was able to refuel postexercise."

Challenges to being vegetarian: "I was low [80–100 grams] in protein; however, upped this intake to around eighteen percent of total calories per day and felt stronger and leaner while competing in my final two ironman races at forty and forty two years old ['94 and '96]."

Alcohol: beer or wine, occasionally a margarita, one time a week

Supplements: PowerBars—three times/day; Vitamin E—800 IU four times per week; Vitamin C—2 grams/day; beta-carotene—25,000 IU/day; iron supplements only three times per week.

Favorite prerace meal: Dave Scott's Pre-Sport Shake (see page 128, chapter 6)

Favorite snacks: PowerBars, walnut bagels, and corn tortillas

9

Plant–Based Diets: Making the Transition

Two women who really bring plant-based diets full circle are Kim Wurzel, member of the U.S. national synchronized swimming team, and Dina Head, WNBA professional basketball player. As All-American athletes competing in technically challenging sports, training two to six hours daily, six days per week, nutrition plays a key role in maintaining their stamina and endurance for thinking and performing.

Kim, a vegan for the last year and a semivegetarian for 6 years, became a complete vegetarian for "health and animal rights." An animal lover, Kim initially became a vegetarian to lose weight. She later eliminated all animal products to "decrease animal cruelty." Her greatest vegetarian challenge mirrors that of other spotlight athletes in the book: finding vegetarian protein sources and enough nutrients in plant-based foods on the road. Even asking the team moms to cook something special is a challenge.In an attempt to replenish her body's needs in a sport that has high-intensity, all-out workouts, Kim consumes a sport bar daily, takes creatine supplements, and eats lots of fruits and saltines for snacks.

Dina, a 28-year-old pesco-vegetarian, also needs to support her training demands. She transformed her low-meat diet in a 2½-year period. She sees the major advantage in being a vegetarian as the elimination of fast foods. With the high demands and wear and tear on her body, ensuring enough protein in her diet is her major challenge. She does a super job on her 109-grams-protein-per-day, 60% carbohydrate diet. On roughly 1,700 calories per day, she is not deficient in any vitamins or minerals. She even enjoys her favorite mainstream snacks of cinnamon grahams, Dole fruit bars, and cinnamon applesauce.

The Plant-Based Transition

Although the transition to a plant-based diet has been relatively easy for the athletes in this book, this is not always the case. In addition to meeting calorie, protein, and vitamin/mineral needs, newly converted vegetarian athletes must find ways to enjoy and thrive without their favorite animal-based products in order to stay on a plant-based diet for peak performance. There are several ways this chapter can help you to do this.

Making the Switch

Like passing the ball to an opponent, the best way to make the switch to plant-based peak-performance eating is by starting today. Take your VSNG nutritional Rx that you calculated from chapters 2 through 5 on energy, carbohydrate, protein, and fat needs and turn to page 190 in this chapter to find the closest VSNG peak performance eating program.

When you find the most appropriate plan, you can adapt the foundation foods and recipes on pages 191–198 to create peak-performance plant-based menus.

Get Radical!

Changing a diet can be a radical event in one's life. Obviously, you've taken the plunge by investing the time to read this book and by preparing your mind and body for plant-based eating. Now that you've seen the research, listened to the testimonials, and assessed the nutrient analysis of the plant-based menus, recipes, and diets of the world-class athletes, you can start your transformation with 100% confidence in meeting your peak performance goals.

Here are some tips to prepare you for preparing the plant-based kitchen:

Purchase the Foundation Foods listed in *The Vegetarian Sports Nutrition Guide* food lists. Then when you make the switch, these foods will be at your fingertips for preparing, serving, and eating the peak-performance recipes and menus from the book.

In addition to the recipes in this book, there are many other vegetarian cookbooks to help you convert familiar recipes, introduce you to the vegetarian world cuisine, and demystify vegetarian basics such as tofu, tempeh, seitan, and soy. There are also many clubs, organizations, and courses you can join to learn more about vegetarianism. These resources are listed in Appendix C.

Remember not to overdo dairy and carbohydrates such as pasta! New vegetarians often make the mistake of overloading on dairy and carbs, getting too many calories and saturated fat and blocking the absorption of iron. They also complain of gaining weight on a vegetarian diet program. Follow *The Vegetarian Sports Nutrition Guide* eating program to get enough but not too much of anything!

Don't be a junk food vegetarian. Yes, candy bars, cookies, jelly beans, and white rice equal a vegetarian diet, but even a vegetarian empty-calorie diet can leave you depleted. Make sure to get variety in all the food groups, including five colors of foods each day: white, brown, red, green, and yellow/orange. These, of course, are not M&M colors!

Check chapter 4 to ensure that you don't get too much protein in your diet. Use the calculations to determine your daily needs. If you feel heavy, dehydrated, or depleted, you may be getting too much protein. Too little protein, and you're bound to lose your hair, break out in pimples, and get sick. Find that perfect daily balance for yourself by using the VSNG food plans in this chapter and adjusting the protein group according to your needs. Remember, you also get protein from the milk alternatives, grains, and vegetable groups.

Look for the best sources of calcium, vitamin B$_{12}$, zinc, and iron if you plan to become animal-free. The best sources of these nutrients are discussed in chapter 7.

Replace the meat in your favorite meals with meat substitutes such as TVP, tempeh, Gimme Lean, and tofu and some prepackaged foods like Boca Burgers, Gardenburgers, Worthington foods, and Morningstar Farms products. Be sure to consider the following:

1. Use soy protein for $\frac{1}{4}$ of the meat in spaghetti sauce, meat loaf, burgers, and sloppy joes.

2. When making tacos and other Mexican delights or casseroles, try half meat, half soy protein.

3. Rather than trying soy sausage or other alternative products by themselves, mix them in soup or a casserole.

4. Try BBQ tofu, grilled tempeh steaks, and meatless cold cuts such as turkey or pastrami. Several fast food chains also offer veggie burgers and meat alternative meals, like Subway's veggie sub (see chapter 10 for other vegetarian fast food choices).

Talk to other vegetarians at my Web site (http://www.lisadorfman. com) or the other Web sites listed in Appendix C of this book.

VEGETARIAN SPORTS NUTRITION GUIDE Food Lists

The Vegetarian Sports Nutrition Guide (VSNG) food lists provide you with a basis for selecting food choices for your daily eating and competing programs.

The VSNG food servings are lists of food portions. They can be compared to similar nutrient contents of the American Dietetic Association and American Diabetes Association food lists for meal planning. Exchange-type lists were initially developed by these organizations to help individuals with diabetes manage blood sugar–related conditions by standardizing the amounts of calories, carbohydrates, proteins, and fats of the six major food groups: milk, protein, vegetables, grains, fruits, and fats.

These *Vegetarian Sports Nutrition Guide* food lists have been adapted to accommodate the nutrient needs of plant-based sports performance diets. The food groups are: protein and meat alternatives, dairy and milk substitutes, vegetables, fruits, fats, and grains/starches. The calorie, carbohydrate, protein, and fat content of each group can be found in the chart on page 190.

These lists of foods highlight the most nutritious food choices, the author's favorite food choices, the VSNG athlete's favorite foods, or are foods included in the recipes throughout the book.

How to use the food lists

▶ Calculate your dietary needs for calories, carbohydrates, protein, and fats.

▶ Look for your personal ideal food plan on page 190.

▶ Look for the amount of food servings you need from each group to achieve peak performance in your sport.

▶ Make selections to achieve the optimal amount of vitamins, minerals, and phytochemicals for peak performance.

▶ Use the menus to design the best daily intake for your personal food program.

▶ You can also include your personal favorite foods. You do this by selecting the most appropriate food group, taking the portion size and calories, and dividing by the calories of that group to get the number of portions from that group.

For instance, you really like this new cookie on the market. One serving has 120 calories. Since it is a grain-based food, you go to the grain list. Each grain serving has 80 calories. Since one serving of your cookies has 120 calories, your cookies are 1.5 portions of grains. If you enjoy three servings of cookies, like most hungry athletes, you have used 4.5 servings of grains.

If you are following the 2,100-calorie VSNG program and you have nine total servings of grain daily, you have used one half of your grain servings on the cookies. This works, but not every day for peak performance! It's better to choose a variety of nutritious foods to be the best you can be.

▲ The Vegetarian Sports Nutrition Eating Program and Food Guide ▼

Food Group/Serving	Pro (gms)	Carb (gms)	Fat (gms)	Energy (Calorie) Levels						
				1,200	1,500	1,800	2,100	2,400	2,700	3,000
Milk or Milk substitutes 100 calories/serving	8	12	varies	2	2	3	3	4	4	4
Fruit 60 calories/serving	0	15	0	4	7	8	8	9	10	14
Vegetables 50 calories/cup	4	10	varies	3 c	3 c	3 c	3 c	3 c	4 c	4 c
Grains/Starches 80 calories/serving	3	15	varies	5	6	8	10	12	14	15
Protein/Meat substitutes 55 calories/serving	7–10	0	varies	3	3	5	6	6	7	8
Fat 45 calories/serving	0	0	5	3	3	3	4	4	4	4
Total calories*:				1,219	1,480	1,856	2,100	2,402	2,717	2,994
Grams/Percentage calories from:										
Carbohydrates				189/62	249/67	306/66	336/64	393/65	448/66	508/68
Protein**				64/21	67/18	95/20	108/21	122/20	139/20	146/20
Fat+				23/17	24/15	28/14	36/15	38/15	41/14	42/12

*Since the calories were calculated using the food servings/exchanges and the Compu-Cal computer, values may not match exact calories for programs designated. Also keep in mind that the calories for each food within each group vary, so if you consistently choose high-calorie foods from that group, your calories will be higher than the plan.

**Although the % of calories from protein appears higher than recommendations from some health care organizations, keep a few thoughts in mind: To decrease protein grams, decrease servings of food from the protein and milk group and increase servings from fruits, fats, and low-protein dairy/dairy substitutes. Remember that when you make these caloric changes, your % of total calories from fat and sugar will increase.

+If you need extra calories or eat in restaurants, at the training table, or on the road often, the proportionately low amount of calories from fat will leave you room for the "extra" that sneaks in during food preparation, baking techniques, and higher-fat sport bars and shakes.

Let's take another example. Your spouse makes great vegetable lasagna with about 290 calories per serving. You don't have the nutritional breakdown, but you know it is made with noodles, low-fat soy cheese, vegetables, and tomato sauce. You can bet it is at least two servings of grains for the noodles (about 1 cup), 1 serving of protein (2 oz) for the low-fat soy cheese, and 1 cup of vegetables for the sauce and veggies. This gives you a total of 160 calories for the grain + 80 calories for the protein + 50 calories for the vegetables, or 290 calories for the slice of lasagna.

If you want to learn more specifically how your favorite recipe fits into your VSNG peak performance eating program, you can fax or e-mail a form like the one at the back of the book to the author's Web site (www.runningnutritionist.com). Your favorite recipe's nutritional analysis and VSNG food servings will be sent to you within 2 to 4 weeks.

▶ VEGETARIAN SPORTS NUTRITION GUIDE Food Groups ◀

Protein and Meat Alternatives
Per serving: about 80 calories, 7–10 grams protein, and variable fat
1 Vegan Original Boca Burger or ¹/₂ Bigger Boca Burger
1 Morningstar Farms Better 'n Burger
³/₄ Gardenburger—Fat Free
4 oz seitan*
1¹/₂ oz White Wave or Lightlife soy tempeh
3 oz Nasoya firm or White Wave Firm tofu
6 oz Mori-Nu lite tofu
2 oz fat-free cheese
1 oz Tofu Rella or Soya Kaas cheese
2 oz fat-free Soya Kaas or Lifetime cheese
³/₄ cup Eggology Egg Whites*
5 egg whites
1 Eggland's Best Egg** (one fat serving)
¹/₂ cup fat-free cottage cheese
2 oz Gimme Lean Meatless ground meat
¹/₄ cup Bob's Red Mill Texturized Vegetable Protein (TVP)

Pesco-vegetarians
2 oz shellfish
2 oz fish
2 oz water-packed tuna

High-Protein Sports Supplements, Bars, and Shakes*

24 oz Optimum Nutrition "Protein Complex—The Drink"
    (2 protein servings)*
High Protein Balance Shake, 1 can—1 protein, 1 starch, 1 fruit serving
1 Met-Rx Shake—2 protein, 1 starch serving
1 Met-Rx Bar—2 protein, 1 milk, 1 starch

*Food fitness note: These are my favorite high-protein food choices after long-distance races, hard strength and endurance training workouts, and several days of consecutive hard workouts. A great way to increase protein grams (some include extra carbs and/or fat).

**The next best thing to the fatless high-protein meal! Eggland's Best Eggs consistently provide less cholesterol (190 vs. 215 mg for ordinary eggs), three times as much Omega-3, 25% Daily Value for Vitamin E (vs. 3%), 40% Daily Value for iodine (vs. 15%), and a higher unsaturated/saturated fat ratio. In addition, their standardized feed formula contains no animal fat, animal byproducts, or processed or recycled foods. They also have weekly testing of feed samples and an on-site USDA inspector.

VSNG Fat Servings

Per serving: approximately 45 calories, 5 grams fat
20 small peanuts
2 tsp peanut butter (1.5 fat servings)
2 tsp Soy Wonder soy nut butter
1 oz Woodstock Farms Dry Roasted Soy Nuts
1/8 medium avocado
2 tbs coconut
1 tbs seeds
1 tsp margarine or butter
1 tsp oil
2 tsp Pataks curry paste
1.5 tbs "Iri Goma" roasted sesame seeds
2 tbs IKARI non-oil sesame dressing (1/4 protein)*

*Deduct this protein serving from your protein food category.

Milk and Milk Substitutes

Per serving: 100 calories, 8 grams protein, 12 grams carbohydrates, variable fat
1 cup soy drink, Fat Free Pacific Vanilla*
1 cup Nutrisoy vanilla lowfat soy milk (1/2 fat)**
1 cup Pacific rice non-fat cocoa drink***
1 cup White Wave Silk chocolate soy beverage****
1 cup Lactaid nonfat milk
1 cup Lactaid 1% fat milk (1/2 fat)
4 oz White Wave flavored soy yogurt
6 oz Organic Vanilla Horizon Yogurt
8 oz container Stonyfield Farms fat-free yogurt (1.5 milk)
3 oz Horizon low-fat sour cream
1 cup non-fat Kefir
1/2 cup Ben & Jerry's Cherry Garcia frozen low-fat yogurt
    (1 milk, 1/2 fat, 1 fruit)

1 Dole frozen pop
1 frozen Tofutti Teddy Fudge Pop—$^3/_4$ milk

*Pacific Vanilla soy drink is fortified with vitamins A and D and calcium.
**Nutrisoy is fortified with vitamins A, D, and B$_2$ and calcium
***Pacific rice drink is fortified with vitamins A and D and calcium
****White Wave Silk chocolate soy beverage is fortified with vitamins A, D, B$_2$, and B$_{12}$ and calcium.

Fruits
Per serving: 60 calories, 15 grams carbohydrates

1 apple, orange, pear, peach, kiwi	15 grapes
$^1/_2$ banana, mango	$^1/_2$ cup cranberries, rhubarb
1 $^1/_4$ cups strawberries, watermelon	1 cup cantaloupe ($^1/_3$ melon)
$^3/_4$ cup pineapple, blueberries	2 plums
1 cup papaya, raspberries	$^3/_4$ cup mandarin oranges

Drinks/juices
1 cup Gatorade
4 oz wine (2 fruits)
$^1/_2$ cup orange, apple, grapefruit, or pineapple juice
$^1/_3$ cup cranberry, prune, or grape juice

Dried Fruits

4 apple rings	1 Go Banana banana
7 apricot halves	$^1/_4$ cup strawberries*
3 prunes	$^1/_4$ cup blueberries*
2 figs	1 date rolled in coconut*
1 oz raisins	

*Available at Wild Oats Grocery Stores, author's guesstimate of portion. No nutritional analysis available.

Other
1 Stretch Island Fruit Leather (1.5 fruits)
1 oz freeze-dried Just Fruit Munchies (2 fruits)
$^1/_2$ cup mixed fresh fruit salad
1 tbs molasses or brown rice syrup
1 tbs jam or jelly

Grains/Starches
Per serving: 80 calories, 15 grams carbohydrates, 2 grams protein, variable fat

Cereals/Grains/Pasta
$^1/_2$ cup bulgur or couscous
Bob's Red Mill 5-grain hot cereal with flaxseed
   ($^1/_3$ cup = 2 grain servings)
$^1/_3$ cup rice
$^1/_2$ cup pasta*

Cereals/Grains/Pasta (*continued*)
Annie Chun's All natural rice noodles (1 oz = $1^1/4$ grain servings)
3 tbs Grape Nuts
3 tbs wheat germ
$^1/2$ cup cooked cereal
$^1/2$ cup shredded wheat
$^1/3$ cup Lifestream Smart Bran
$^1/2$ cup Lifestream Flax Plus
$^1/2$ cup Coco O's
1 Barbara's Toaster Pastry (like Pop Tart) (2 servings grain and $^1/2$ fruit)
1 Flax Plus Waffle (1 serving plus $^1/2$ protein)
Boboli Bread Stick—1 stick (1 starch, $^1/2$ protein)
German Bread Haus—Wheat and Yeast Free Power Bread—
    1 slice (1 starch, $^1/2$ fat)

*Try a variety of pastas, including Hudson Mills Whole Wheat spirals, Vita Spelt, Ancient Harvest Quinoa, Sobaya organic wheat and brown rice "soba" pasta, and buckwheat "soba" pasta. Quinoa pasta is rich in vitamins B_1 and B_2, soba pasta in iron, whole wheat pasta in vitamins B_1 and B_3.

Bread/Crackers
Natural Crispbread Bible Bread—2 crackers
$^1/2$ bagel
7 Japanese Umenokamaki Rice Crackers
25 Eden sea vegetable or wasabi crackers
1 piece JJ Flats (1.5 servings) (variety of flavors including poppy seed
    and sesame)
1 whole wheat pita, small
$^1/2$ whole wheat pita, large
1 flour tortilla (1.5 servings)
1 corn tortilla
1 Alvarado Street sprouted wheat tortilla ($^1/2$ protein serving)
2" × 2" piece Grainaissance Mochi ($1^1/2$ starch)
38 Papadum Lentil Chips

Chips/Snack Foods/Rice Cakes
"8 Mate," Assorted rice cracker with green peas snack* ($1^1/4$ starch
    servings, $^1/2$ fat)
9 Tree of Life jalapeño rice cakes**
8 Baked Lay's potato chips
1.5 large rice cakes
8 mini Quaker Rice Cakes
5 Hain Mini Rice Cakes
17 Hain Cookie Jar Rice Cake Bits*
1 oz Bruno and Luigi's Pasta Chips ($^1/4$ protein)
1 large hard Snyder's pretzel ($1^1/4$ grains)

7 Shiloh Farms Oat Bran Pretzels
Ana Hana Brand—Snack Bean Party Mix "IMOTO"
     (1 starch, $^1/_2$ protein, $^1/_2$ fat)

*Available at Asian food stores.
**Comes in other flavors; my favorite is jalapeño.

Starchy Vegetables
Potato—1 baked or $^1/_2$ cup Barbara's mashed
$^1/_2$ cup corn
$^1/_2$ cup peas
$^1/_3$ cup yams
$^3/_4$ cup winter squash (spaghetti, acorn, butternut)

Beans and Bean Products
$^1/_2$ cup Eden's garbanzo beans
$^1/_2$ cup fava or lima beans
$^1/_3$ cup pinto beans
$^1/_2$ cup Westbrae Natural Soybeans (2 protein, 2 fat, 1 grain)
2 tbs Fantastic Foods Hummus
$^1/_4$ cup Fantastic Foods Instant Refried Beans
$^1/_2$ cup Shari's Refried Beans ($^1/_2$ protein)

Other
3 tsp arrowroot ($^1/_2$ grain serving)

Combination Foods
1 Mrs. T's Pierogie
1 package Amy's black beans, vegetables enchilada (2 starches, 1 protein)
Amy's Organic Beans and Rice Burrito (2 grains, $^1/_2$ protein, 1 fat)
1 container dried Health Valley Chili (2 veg, 1 protein, 1 grain)
     or 1 can (2 proteins, 2 starch, 1 cup veggies)
Amy's Roasted Vegetable Pizza—No cheese, 1 pizza pie (2 starch,
     1 protein, $^1/_2$ fat)

Beverages
1 beer (2 grains)
1 lite beer (1$^1/_2$ grains)
1 cup Amazake rice drink (2 starches)

Sweets
8 pieces Red Panda licorice
3 sticks Bearitos black licorice or 2.5 sticks red
1 Home Yokan-Japanese cookie (1 grain, 2.5 fruits)
1 Japanese Sanshoku Dango rice cake (actually rice-covered bean-filled
     sweet dumplings) (1 starch)
$^1/_8$ of entire prepared pie crust (1 fat)
1 Imagine Pudding Cup (2 servings)

Sweets *(continued)*
American Licorice Co. Cocoa, Orange,
   or Licorice Herbal Chews (1 starch, 1 fruit)
4 pieces Soken Natural Seaweed Candy (no simple sugars)
20 pieces Sunspire Natural Chocolate Candy (1 fat)
1 Häagen-Dazs Chocolate Sorbet Bar
2 Tofutti Chocolate Fudge Treats

Sport Bars
1 Ironman Bar (1 starch, 1 1/4 protein, 1 fat)
1 Prozone or Balance Bar (1 starch, 1 protein, 1 fat)
1 PowerBar (1 starch, 1 protein, 1 fruit, 1/2 fat)
1 Ultrafuel Bar (1 starch, 1 protein, 1 fruit)
1 Clif Bar (1 starch, 1 protein, 1 fruit, 1/2 fat)
1 Mountain Lift Bar (1 starch, 1 protein, 1 fruit)
1 You Are What You Eat Bar (2 starch, 1 fruit)

Vegetables
Per cup: 50 calories, 10 grams carbohydrates, 4 grams protein

eggplant	asparagus
broccoli	artichoke
kale	onions
cauliflower	squash—zucchini
carrots	radishes
cabbage	celery
brussels sprouts	mung bean sprouts
mushrooms	snow peas
peppers—red, yellow,	tomato sauce—fat free
orange, green	bok choy
okra	other greens: spinach, collard
tomatoes	vegetable juice

Other
hot Just Veggies (1/2 cup)

Free Foods
To complement your vegetarian meals. These foods have negligible calories.

lettuce	soy sauce
garlic	mustard
watercress	chili sauce
onions	Guiltless Gourmet Salsa
lemons	Coffee, tea, or sparkling
limes	unsweetened water
jalapeño	

▶ THE VEGETARIAN SPORTS NUTRITION GUIDE ◀
Recipe Food Servings

RECIPE	PROTEIN	GRAINS	VEGETABLES (CUPS)	FRUITS	MILK	FAT
Hanners' Tempeh Gumbo	0	3.0	1.25	0	0	1.0
Hanners' Fava Bean Hummus	0	1.0	0	0	0	0
Hanners' Hummus	0	2.5	0	0	0	0
Hanners' Vegetarian Chili	1.5	0	2.5	0	0	0
Hanners' Phyto Veggie Explosion	0.5	1.5	2.0	0.5	0	0
Hanners' Roasted Eggplant Pomodoro	0	0	3.0	0	0	1.0
Hanners' Rice and Red Beans	0.5	6.0	0	0	0	0
Hanners' Apple Tower Dessert	0	1.5	0	1.5	0	1.0
Stephens' No Horsing Around Veggie Plate	0	5.5	1.75	0	0	0
Mathews' Marathon BBQ Tempeh	0	1.5	0	0	0	1.0
Wurzel and Mathews' Marathon Prerace Pasta Blaster	0	4.0	1.0	0	0	0
Brown's Curling Key Lime Pie	0	1.5	0	0	0.5	1.0
Brown's Curling Kenyan Tortilla	0	4.0	3.5	0	0	2.5
Brown's Curling Combo	0	3.5	0	2.0	1.0	0
Didonato's Swimming Rice Primavera	0	6.0	1.0	0	0	1.0
Dave Scott's Pre-Sport Shake	0.5	0	0	3.5	1.0	1.0
Ruth's Ironwoman Pho	1.5	1.5	0	0	0	0
Ruth's PR Porridge	0	3.0	1.0	1.5	0	0
Charlene's Triple Axel Veggie Surprise	2.0	2.0	1.0	0	0	1.5
Heath's Skating Mexican Fiesta Meal	0	4.0	0.25	0	0	3.0
Abate's Minestrone	0	3.0	2.0	0	0	0
Still's "Defensive" Stir-Fry	0	0	4.0	0	0	0.5
Welzel's Indian CousCous	0	4.0	3.0	0	0	1.0
Slam Dunk Fish Dish	3.5	0	1.0	0	0	5.0
Dina's Prehoop Meal	4.0	4.0	2.5	0	0	2.0
Stephens' No Horsing Around Precompetition Snack	0	0.5	0	0.5	0	2.0
Charlene's Skating Supplement	0	0	0	1.0	0	1.0
Charlene's Skating Supplement w/oats	0	2.0	0	0	0	1.0

RECIPE	PROTEIN	GRAINS	VEGETABLES (CUPS)	FRUITS	MILK	FAT
Charlene's Skating Supplement w/OJ "Smooth Sailing" Prerace Meal	0	0	0	1.0	0	1.0
Lisa's Bean Taco Pie	1.0	2.0	0.5	0	0	0
Lisa's Scrambled Whites and Greens (peas)	2.0	1.5	0	0	0	0
Scrambled Whites with Spinach/Mushrooms	4.0	0	1.0	0	0	0
Lisa's Field of Greens w/Soy Cheese	1.5	0.5	2.5	0	0	0

Dina's Prehoop Meal

Makes 1 serving*

———

$3\frac{1}{2}$ servings salmon

1 cup mixed frozen vegetables

2 cups brown rice

———

Prepare salmon by baking at 375°F for 10–15 minutes. Prepare brown rice according to package. Steam mixed vegetables.

▶ Nutrients per serving: 725 calories, 41 grams protein, 115 grams carbohydrate, 11 grams fat, 1 gram monounsaturated fat, 1 gram linoleic fat, 7 grams fiber

▶ Dietary composition: 23% protein, 64% carbohydrates, 14% fat

▶ VSNG food servings: 2.5 cups vegetables, 4 grains, 4 protein, 2 fats

▶ Good source of vitamin A, B_1, B_3, D, potassium, phosphorus, magnesium, manganese, selenium; moderate source of vitamin B_2, B_6, pantothenic acid, iron, zinc

*Food fitness note: Dina needs her strength for four basketball periods, but other athletes can share the dish with a friend to reduce calories and other nutrients.

▶ THE VEGETARIAN SPORTS NUTRITION GUIDE ◀
Peak Performance 14-Day Training Menus

Note: Adapt your calorie level and servings to the recommended meals below. Include 7–9 cups fluids daily including water, green tea, sport drink, and/or wine and beer. Include enough fluids, vegetables, salads, and fruits to meet your energy needs.

	DAY 1 MENU	DAY 2 MENU
Morning	Ben's Laser Oats, dried or fresh banana	Ruth's PR Porridge
Snack	Parillo Bar	Melon and dried fruit
Afternoon	Fruit salad w/soy or frozen yogurt	Ruth's Ironwoman Pho, Eden's Hot 'n Spicy Wasabi Chips
Snack	Shiloh Farms oat bran pretzels	Guiltless Gourmet Chips and Salsa
Evening	Stephens' No Horsing Around Veggie Plate, baked potato	Didonato's Rice Primavera
Snack	Popcorn	Häagen-Dazs pop or Tofutti pop

	DAY 3 MENU	DAY 4 MENU
Morning	Brown's Curling Combo with WestSoy Plus	Dave Scott's Pre-Sport Shake
Snack	Fruit smoothie	Rice crackers with apple and Soya Kaas cheese
Afternoon	Abate's Minestrone, tossed green salad, whole grain rolls	Hanners' Vegetarian Chili, Guiltless Gourmet Chips
Snack	Raisins and soy nuts	Dole fruit pop
Evening	Amy's Bean and Rice Burrito	Mathews' BBQ Tempeh
Snack	Hain's Cookie Jar rice cake bits	Japanese rice cake

	DAY 5 MENU	DAY 6 MENU
Morning	Whole wheat bagel with strawberry jam, fresh fruit salad	Eggology whites scrambled w/greens
Snack	PowerBar's Protein Plus Bar	Strawberries and cream
Afternoon	Lisa's Field of Greens w/Miso Dressing, rice crackers	Boca Burger w/Soy Cheese on whole wheat bun
Snack	banana, dates and figs, fresh apple	Cinnamon applesauce
Evening	Welzel's Marathon Couscous	Wurzel and Mathews' Marathon Prerace Pasta Blaster
Snack	Red Panda licorice	Imagine Pudding Cup

DAY 7 MENU

Morning	Old Savannah flapjacks with natural fruit syrup
Snack	Starbucks' Power Drink
Afternoon	Amy's Burrito
Snack	Citrus fruit
Evening	Hanners' Rice and Red Beans
Snack	Glass of wine or Ame*

DAY 8 MENU

Strawberry or blueberry fruit smoothie

Fresh strawberries and cream

Barbara's mashed potatoes and green peas

Frozen protein fruit smoothie

Joe's Bearito Taco Shell w/beans, salsa, lettuce, and tomato

Health Nut cookies

DAY 9 MENU

Morning	High Protein Balance Shake, fresh fruit
Snack	Raisin-cinnamon mochi and green tea
Afternoon	Lisa's Bean Taco Pie
Snack	Trail mix, Stretch Island fruit rollup
Evening	Hanners' Phyto Veggie Explosion
Snack	Quaker Mini Flavored Rice Cakes

DAY 10 MENU

Ben' Cheerios/Grape-Nuts mix

Fresh mango or papaya

Baked potato w/broccoli and melted soy cheese

Häagen-Dazs yogurt/sorbet bar

Spaghetti w/Hanners' Roasted Eggplant Pomodoro

Popcorn, American Licorice Company's Orange Herbal Chews

DAY 11 MENU

Morning	Jane's Mocha espresso w/toasted mochi
Snack	Apple and Soya Kaas cheese
Afternoon	Fat-free cottage cheese and berries
Snack	You Are What You Eat Bar
Evening	Gardenburger on whole-grain bun w/lettuce and tomato
Snack	Ice cream w/Japanese cookie

DAY 12 MENU

Craig's Granola w/raisins and fat-free Lactaid or soy milk

Stoker bar

Lisa's Field of Greens and jalapeño fat-free soy cheese

Sweet potato

Charlene's Triple Axel Veggie Surprise

Ginger/shoya tea, Brown's Curling Key Lime Pie

	DAY 13 MENU	DAY 14 MENU
Morning	Scrambled Eggology w/peas	Buckwheat waffles w/strawberries and cream
Snack	Walnut bagel	Watermelon
Afternoon	Hanners' Hummus w/whole wheat pita	Subway's veggie sub on whole wheat roll
Snack	Cinnamon grahams	Parillo Bar
Evening	Hanners' Tempeh Gumbo, organic greens	Brown's Curling Kenyan Tortilla
Snack	Frozen sorbet or rice-based frozen dessert	Hanners' Apple Tower Dessert

*sparkling non-alcoholic fruit juice and herb blend

Spotlight Athlete

Dina Head

WNBA basketball player

Age: 27

2 years semivegetarian

Alcohol: none

Supplements: vitamin B_{12}, C, E

Reason for becoming vegetarian: "No particular reason . . . change of pace and basically a natural change over the past two and half years."

Advantages of being vegetarian: "Eliminates all of the bad foods like fast food."

Challenges to being vegetarian: "Making sure you get enough protein, especially with the high demands and wear and tear on your body."

Favorite pregame meal: Head's Pre-Hoop Fish Dish (page 198)

Favorite snacks: cinnamon grahams, cinnamon applesauce, Dole fruit bars

Favorite one-pot meal: Head's Slam Dunk Fish Dish (page 102)

▲ The Vegetarian Sports Nutrition Guide Recipe Analysis Summary ▼

Recipe	Chapter	Calories	Carbohy-drates (gms)	Protein (gms)	Fat (gms)	Phyto chemicals?	Vitamins/minerals*
Hanners' Tempeh Gumbo	6	340	55	13	8	Y	folate, K, potassium, magnesium
Hanners' Fava Bean Hummus	4	97	17	4	1	Y	C, potassium, manganese
Hanners' Hummus	1	217	36	11	3	Y	potassium, phosphorus, iron
Hanners' Vegetarian Chili	3	333	46	24	8	Y	A, C, folate, K, potassium, iron
Hanners' Phyto Veggie Explosion	7	297	60	17	1	Y	A, C, K, folate, sodium, potassium
Hanners' Roasted Eggplant Pomodoro	1	213	39	7	7	Y	A, C, folate, potassium, K
Hanners' Rice and Red Beans	3	466	93	15	4	Y	
Hanners' Apple Tower Dessert	10	402	90	4	5	N	manganese
Stephens' No Horsing Around Veggie Plate	7	466	97	18	4	Y	B_1, B_3, B_6, A, C, E, K, sodium, potassium, selenium, phosphorus, manganese
Mathews' Marathon BBQ Tempeh	4	246	29	19	7	Y	
Wurzel and Mathews' Marathon Prerace Pasta Blaster	3	344	65	14	2	Y	B_1, B_2, iron
Brown's Curling Key Lime Pie	10	206	36	5	5	N	
Brown's Curling Kenyan Tortilla	5	570	96	24	13	Y	A, C, B_3, B_6, folate, K, phosphorus, iron, copper
Brown's Curling Combo	10	439	93	17	2	N	A, B_1, B_2, B_3, B_6, B_{12}, K, phosphorus
Didonato's Swimming Rice Primavera	5	493	95	17	7	Y	A, B_1, B_6, K, folate, biotin, pantothenic acid, phosphorus, potassium, manganese, iron
Dave Scott's Pre-Sport Shake	6	363	62	13	9	Y	B_6, folate, C,
Ruth's Ironwoman Pho	7	244	43	14	2	Y	A, C, B_1, B_2, B_3, B_6, folate, E, K, pantothenic acid, phosphorus, manganese

Recipe	Chapter	Calories	Carbohydrates (gms)	Protein (gms)	Fat (gms)	Phyto chemicals?	Vitamins/minerals*
Ruth's PR Porridge	2	408	90	9	3	Y	A, C, E, B$_6$, K, magnesium, selenium, manganese
Charlene's Triple Axel Veggie Surprise	5	332	34	22	15	Y	A, magnesium, manganese, iron
Heath's Skating Mexican Fiesta Meal	5	485	63	19	19	Y	K, folate, iron
Abate's Deca-Minestrone	4	335	65	19	2	Y	A, B$_6$, C, K, iron
Still's "Defensive" Stir-Fry	4	214	38	14	5	Y	A, C, K, folate, pantothenic acid, potassium
Welzel's Marathon Couscous	3	470	90	25	5	Y	A, C, B$_6$, K, folate, selenium, manganese, potassium
Slam Dunk Fish Dish	5	361	8	27	25	N	C, K, B$_{12}$, folate, chloride
Dina's Prehoop Meal	9	725	115	41	11	Y	A, B$_1$, B$_3$ D, K, phosphorus, magnesium, manganese, selenium
Stephens' No Horsing Around Skating Precompetition Snack	10	148	17	2	9	N	K
Charlene's Skating Supplement	8	8	8	2	7	N	folate
Charlene's Skating Supplement w/oats	8	231	33	8	9	Y	B$_1$, folic acid, phosphorus, manganese
Charlene's Skating Supplement w/OJ	8	142	21	3	7	Y	B$_1$, folate, C, phosphorus
Ben's "Smooth Sailing" Prerace Meal	3	490	66	39	7	Y	E, phosphorus, magnesium, selenium
Lisa's Bean Taco Pie	3	255	41	17	3	Y	C, folate, iron
Lisa's Scrambled Whites and Greens (peas)	4	183	13	30	0	N	K
Scrambled Whites with Spinach/Mushrooms	4	2	6	54	0	Y	K
Lisa's Field of Greens w/Soy Cheese	10	291	33	33	5	Y	A, C, K, folate, potassium, iron

*Indicates vitamins and minerals in amounts above 50% RDAs. Other vitamins and minerals are listed with recipes.

Kim Wurzel

U.S. national synchronized swimming team

Age: 21

5 years vegetarian, 1 year vegan

Reason for becoming vegetarian: "For health and cruelty reasons. I first stopped eating all red meat, fish, and pork because I was told I needed to watch my weight. Then, a year ago, I decided I didn't like the fact that I was eating an animal. I am an animal lover and I hate seeing cruelty to animals. It makes me feel like I am helping the animals by not eating them."

Challenges to being vegetarian: "Being in a sport that has high-intensity workouts, it's difficult to get all that I need to replenish my body. I need to be aware of not getting enough protein and nutrients that meat has. It's also hard when we go to competitions and there are not a lot of choices to eat. We have team mothers cook for us and it's difficult to always ask them to make me something special. I try not to be a difficult person, but I will not eat meat."

Supplements: creatine powder and PowerBars

Favorite premeet meal: pasta with marinara sauce and vegetables

Favorite snacks: fruits and saltine crackers

10

Competition Time: Plant-Based Diets in Action

Now that you've had a chance to make the transition to a plant-based eating program, applied your personal nutrition prescription for training into an eating program, and maybe had a chance to taste some of the athletes' favorite recipes and snacks, it's time to learn how to handle those special moments in an athlete's life.

The Vegetarian Sports Nutrition Guide has given you a solid sports science foundation, and now you're ready to address some of the more challenging times. The VSNG athletes have identified these times as being on the road, losing weight for peak performance and for pre-competition periods of carbo-loading and making weight, and the postrecovery period.

Whether they're training or competing, the two Olympic-level athletes spotlighted in this chapter understand the nutritional demands of their sports and the ideal competitive state that's required for their best mental and physical performance.

Erika Brown is a talented former University of Wisconsin Academic All Big Ten MVP golfer who went on to compete in Olympic curling and represent the United States for the first time in Nagano, Japan. Now 26, Erika has been a lacto-ovo-vegetarian for 9 years. She eliminated meat from her Midwestern diet for health and ethical reasons. In addition to feeling more energized, healthy, and active, she knows she is making an environmental contribution. "People take notice when they find out I'm vegetarian and with any luck take a closer look at their diets."

Debbie Stephens, an Olympic-level equestrian show jumper, "just wanted to lose weight and be more energetic!" As a pesco-vegetarian for 19 years, Debbie's only challenge is finding food at competitions. Erika agrees that finding healthy nonanimal protein sources in small Midwestern meat-and-potatoes towns is also her "good lesson in planning ahead!"

As discussed in chapter 3, eating prior to competition is a challenge. For all the training hours an athlete invests before the big event, it can be ruined with just one bad meal. You have learned the formulas for calculating your precompetition carbohydrate needs, fluid requirements, and other guidelines, but *what* exactly do you eat? Some of these performance-breaking issues will be discussed in this chapter.

Special Diets

The vegetarian athlete has already selected a special diet to meet his or her needs. If you read the popular press, you know that there have been many controversies recently regarding the proportion of calories an athletic person needs from carbohydrates, proteins, and fats. Others have been told to fast or adopt other dietary techniques that may actually hinder performance. Here are some of those programs.

Losses and Gains

You've learned so much about calculating your dietary needs based on your present weight. What if the plant-based athlete wants to lose weight or fat or even gain weight?

In chapter 4, the protein needs of strength athletes were discussed. A prescription of 1.4 to 1.8 grams of protein per kilogram body weight per day was advised. To increase muscle mass, an additional 28 grams per day was suggested. However, in order for protein to be used to build muscle mass, substantial amounts of calories must be consumed. In order to calculate the most appropriate calorie intake, you must calculate your energy needs based on your desirable weight.

If your goal is to lose weight and body fat, the following formula can help you calculate your desirable body weight.

To calculate the appropriate weight for your desired percent body fat, take the following steps:

Get your fat weight.

Fat weight = current weight × (current % body fat)
For example: 150-pound athlete × .15 (15% body fat)
= 22.5 pounds body fat

Calculate your lean body weight (LBW).

Lean body weight = current weight − fat weight
150-pound athlete − 22.5 pounds fat weight
= 127.5 pounds lean body weight

Then, using the values from steps one and two, select your goal percent body fat composition.

For example: 150-pound athlete desires 10% body fat

To calculate approximate weight goal for your desired body fat goal, take your lean body weight and divide by 1 − (% body fat desired).

For 150-pound athlete with 127.5 pounds lean body weight,
divided by 1 −.10 (.90)
Desired body weight = 127.5 divided by .90 = 142 pounds

This athlete would need to lose approximately 8 pounds of fat weight to meet his desired percentage of body fat goal of 10%. Now try the formula with your own weight and desired percentage of body fat goal.

In order to decrease 8 pounds of fat, the athlete could

▶ Decrease his total dietary calories no more than 500 calories per day. The ideal way to do this is to cut out excess sugars and fats.

▶ Increase his energy expenditure through aerobic and anaerobic exercise.

Fasting

Athletes who need to achieve rapid weight loss and/or improve athletic performance sometimes use fasting. Fasting can be detrimental to physical and psychological performance.

After the first day of fasting, liver glycogen is depleted. In order for the body to maintain blood sugar, it breaks down muscle to supply glucogenic amino acids. After a week of fasting, muscle contributes about one-third of the weight loss. This is undesirable for the competitive athlete and can contribute to other problems.

Fasting also causes the body's metabolism to slow down and reduces the BEE (discussed in chapter 1). This means that it will take fewer calories to fuel the athlete at the present weight. With fewer calories consumed, often vitamins and minerals will be sacrificed. Hence, the athlete will start to feel run down. In addition, since most of the weight loss is water weight, critical electrolytes, discussed in chapters 6 and 8, will also be lost. That can impair muscle and kidney function.

At worst, the athlete can get severe headaches, feel lightheaded, and get nauseous and possibly pass out, a real danger to the cyclist training in the city. This is due to the ketosis and acidosis (acidic pH in the blood) that results from the lack of carbohydrates needed for the brain and central nervous system.

Weight Gain

It may be even more difficult for an underweight athlete to gain one pound than for an overweight athlete to lose one pound. The best way to gain weight on a plant-based diet is to add an additional 500 calories per day to your VSNG Peak Performance Nutrition Formula.

Other eating and training suggestions include

▶ Decreasing training if overtrained, undernourished, and glycogen-depleted (see chapter 3)

▶ Following protein recommendations for strength athletes, with a minimum of 100 grams of protein per day

▶ Eating within 1 hour before working out so the body uses energy from the food consumed and not from stored sources

▶ Adding nutrient-dense, high-carbohydrate foods with added fats such as soy margarine or sauces (see Hanners' Roasted Eggplant Pomodoro on page 25) or by consuming an extra high-calorie, high-protein sport bar or sport shake at snack time, such as Met-Rx

There are many other shakes, powders, and potions devoted to this on the market. Including them at mealtime or snack time may help by taking the thinking out of food planning. You may just want to make a batch of Dave Scott's Pre-Sport Shake and add Charlene's Skating Supplement to achieve the same results.

Among the most popular supplements advertised to enhance muscle mass are chromium, creatine, vanadium, boron, beta-hydroxy-beta-methylbutyrate (HMB), protein, and amino acids. Some of these supplements were discussed in chapter 8. An outline of these in regard to increasing muscle mass and weight gain is contained in the following table.

▶ Summary of Supplements Promoted for Weight Gain ◀

SUPPLEMENT	CLAIM	SAFETY AND/OR EFFECTIVENESS
Chromium	Increases lean body mass	Not effective; can accumulate in cells and cause chromosomal damage
Creatine	Increases muscle mass	Even though its safety was questioned when wrestlers died from supplementation, it was found that they were on dangerous dehydration programs that led to their deaths; long-term use has not been examined; short-term use (described in chapter 8) has shown beneficial and positive effects; a side effect may be enhanced anaerobic performance and perhaps water weight gain
Vanadium	Anabolic effects	Could have detrimental effects; larger doses than 13.5 mg/day for 6 weeks or 9 mg/day up to 16 months can cause diarrhea, green tongue, cramps, and GI problems; not recommended
Boron	Increases testosterone and muscle mass	No effects in one study with male bodybuilders; questionable
HMB	Prevents protein breakdown to increase muscle mass	Possibly effective (see chapter 8), but not dramatic; further studies are needed
Amino acids (AA)	Stimulate growth hormone, increase body mass, decrease fat	Arginine, orthinine, histidine, lysine, methionine, and phenylalanine major AAs promoted; most supplements contain less AA than 4 grams ($\frac{1}{2}$ oz protein); taking specific AAs can cause imbalances, cramps, and diarrhea

40/30/30

This program recommends a nutrient breakdown of 40% of calories from carbohydrates, 30% from protein, and 30% from fat. This diet has been recommended for weight and fat loss for better performance. Some advocates of this program sell bars, drinks, and pills to enhance the benefits.

In a nutshell, if you compare this diet to a high-carbohydrate, moderate-protein, low-fat program encouraged by research throughout the book, it just doesn't jive. The 40/30/30 program can potentially leave the athlete glycogen-depleted, protein-overdosed, and on the border of too much fat. A visit to the local restaurant on the wrong day can mean an extra 14 grams of fat from a tablespoon of oil added to the chef's best blackened fish special or grilled veggies. It's just too close for comfort.

In the brochure *Questioning 40/30/30, A Guide to Understanding Sports Nutrition Advice,* a comparison of the 40/30/30 program and the high-carbohydrate diet program discussed throughout this book would look like this for the 70-kg athlete:

▶ Comparison of a High-Carbohydrate Diet ◀ to 40/30/30

NUTRIENT	RECOMMENDED 65/15/20	40/30/30	COMMENTS
Calories	3,500	3,500	OK
Carbohydrates (gms)	570 (8 g/kg)	350 (5 g/kg)	low
Protein (gms)	131 (1.9 g/kg)	350 (5 g/kg)	high
Fat (gms)	78	117	high

Adapted from *40/30/30* brochure.

Losing Weight on 40/30/30

Since carbohydrates are demanded and recommended for high-intensity and long-distance exercise, this program would not be as beneficial as the high-carbohydrate diet for these events. Since there is no special diet for burning more fat other than some training and eating techniques described in chapter 5, this program will probably not help the average athlete use more fat for energy as promoted. And if the athlete is glycogen-depleted, he will not be able to fuel himself by using fat when the time comes. So on a theoretical basis alone, 40/30/30 cannot be recommended as the best program for sports training.

On the Other Hand

As always, there is another side to all of this. If the athlete eats a very poor high-sugar, low-nutrient, high-carbohydrate diet, she is probably not feeling or performing her best. She may feel sluggish, be holding extra water from the abundance of low-fiber, high-simple-carbohydrate diet of muffins, bagels, sport bars, drinks, and sweets, and be ready for a change. The 40/30/30 plan would rescue her from this dull existence. The higher-protein, lower-carbohydrate intake can help her to eliminate some of that edema accumulated from the excess carbohydrate intake, possibly manage her blood sugar by controlling her simple, high-glycemic sugar intake, and help her consume a better balance of nutrients at every meal.

Even though none of the VSNG athletes ascribes to this plan, Charlene has alluded to needing higher-fat, less sugary foods in her program to manage her mood and energy levels. Indeed, the plant-based athlete interested in the 40/30/30 plan can modify the VSNG food guide to create a more 40/30/30–like program without sacrificing the goodness of the VSNG food package.

To create a 40/30/30 plant-based peak performance program, the VSNG athlete can

- ▶ choose a sport bar for snacks that meets a 40/30/30 profile, like Balance or PR Bars
- ▶ eat regular popcorn, chips, and even trail mix for higher-fat snacks instead of fruit and grains
- ▶ include more protein servings from seitan, tofu, and Eggology egg whites and fewer grain servings (each portion is equivalent in calories, so just switch one for one)
- ▶ allot your VSNG food portions to provide a 40/30/30 balance of food at every meal

Precompetition Meals

This area of sports science, already discussed in chapter 3, has been getting a tremendous amount of attention in recent years. It is evident from the abundance of sport bars, gels, drinks, and shakes on the market. The demand for fuel prior to competition has been validated and has gone far beyond the cola-and-candy-bar prerace jolt. Despite this, some athletes like Debbie still enjoy a candy bar and coffee before their big event.

Many of the athletes have special preferences for the prerace evening meal. Some of their favorite choices include pasta, cereals, pancakes, and sport bars. Their favorite prerace meals can be found on page 45.

The market for precompetition meals has also extended into competition foods. Since it is difficult to run or cycle with a plate of pasta or swim with a sport shake, a new line of sport gels has emerged. These gels are easy to eat, digest, and store; small and portable; and a no-frills source of carbohydrates. As discussed in chapter 3, carbohydrates are an ideal source of energy for long-distance or high-intensity work. These high-carbohydrate sport gels provide a variety of sugars, primarily simple, and sometimes include the addition of vitamins, minerals, caffeine, branched chain amino acids, and buffering agents. As with bars and drinks, always try these during training so you know which one works best for you. Since these products are also deficient in fluid, you need to drink up when consuming these sugar packets. A summary of some of the gels is found on page 215. High-performance sports drinks and beverages can be found listed in chapter 6.

Stephens' No Horsing Around Precompetition Snack

1 oz candy bar*
1 cup brewed coffee

I know what you're thinking, but see the food fitness note!

▶ Nutrients per serving: 148 calories, 2 grams protein, 17 grams carbohydrates, 9 grams fat, 5 grams saturated fat, 14 grams sugar

▶ Dietary composition: 6% protein, 43% carbohydrates, 52% fat

▶ VSNG food servings: $\frac{1}{2}$ grain, $\frac{1}{2}$ fruit, 2 fats

▶ Good source of vitamin K

*Food fitness note: I know what you're thinking! Actually, this was a favorite prerace meal for several of my top-level racing friends from the 1980s (before the days of sport bars). The candy bar does provide sugar and caffeine for an energy boost.

Brown's Curling Pre-Meet Combo

Makes 1 serving

$\frac{1}{2}$ cup Cheerios cereal*

$\frac{1}{2}$ cup Grape Nuts cereal*

1 cup skim milk*

1 banana

Eat in large bowl.

▶ Nutrients per serving: 439 calories, 17 grams protein, 93 grams carbohydrate, 2 grams fat, 32 grams sugar, 5 grams fiber

▶ Dietary composition: 15% protein, 81% carbohydrates, 4% fat

▶ VSNG food servings: 1 milk, 2 fruits, 3.5 grains

▶ Good source of vitamin A, B_1, B_2, B_3, B_6, B_{12}, folate, potassium, phosphorus; moderate source of calcium, magnesium, iron, sodium, vitamin C, pantothenic acid

*Food fitness note: You can choose a variety of low-sugar, low-fiber cereals. Read the labels and find cereals that contain less than 5 grams of sugar. I also recommend fat-free Lactaid milk, fat-free soy milk, or fat-free rice milk for competition morning.

▶ Sport Gels for Precompetition ◀

GEL NAME	CARBOHYDRATE SOURCE	CALORIES	COMMENTS
Clif Shot	brown rice syrup	198/tube	various flavors; chocolate espresso has caffeine, sodium, potassium, and ginseng; has a good, natural rich taste
Power Gel	maltodextrin, fructose	110/pack	various flavors; sodium, potassium, antioxidants, caffeine, and ginseng added; sweet taste, easy to carry
Gu	maltodextrin, fructose	100/pack	antioxidants, potassium, sodium, calcium, and ginseng added; easy to carry, thick consistency
Gatorade ReLode	maltodextrin, dextrose	80/pack	salt and potassium added; very easy to transport
Squeezy	maltodextrin, fructose	80/pack	very easy to transport; various flavors, simple formula
Jog Mate	milk sugar	100/tube	encouraged as a postexercise gel, although appropriate for long-distance events; great taste; 10 grams protein, vitamin- and mineral-fortified

Note: Remember that your body has an hourly limit on the amount of carbohydrates it can metabolize per hour. More than about 75 grams can make your belly play Beethoven's Fifth if you overdo the sugars from sport drinks, bars, and gels.

Carbohydrate Loading

Ideal for long-distance sports such as the marathon and ironman, this eating/training regimen begins one week prior to an event to maximize glycogen stores and is discussed in greater detail in chapter 3. This section includes the VSNG guide to food servings for 1,200 to 3,000 calories for the carbo-loading regimen and the menus to assist you in making the best meal choices.

► Carbo–Loading Phase: Peak Performance on Plant-Based Diets ▼

Food Group/Serving	Pro (gms)	Carb (gms)	Fat (gms)	Energy (Calorie) Levels — Daily Food Servings						
				1,200	1,500	1,800	2,100	2,400	2,700	3,000
Milk or Milk substitutes 100 calories/serving	8	12	varies	1	1	2	3	3	4	4
Fruit 60 calories/serving		15		6	8	8	9	11	12	15
Vegetables 50 calories/cup	4	10	varies	3 c	3 c	3 c	3 c	3 c	3 c	3 c
Grains/Starches 80 calories/serving	3	15	varies	6	7	9	11	12	14	15
Protein/Meat substitutes 55 calories/serving	7–10		varies	3	4	5	6	7	8	8
Fat 45 calories/serving			5	1	1	1	1	2	2	2
Total calories				1,250	1,488	1,767	2,106	2,389	2,728	2,989
Grams/% calories from:										
Carbohydrates*				222/71	267/72	309/70	366/70	411/70	468/70	528/71
Protein				59/19	69/19	90/20	111/21	121/20	142/20	145/19
Fat**				14/10	16/9	19/10	22/9	29/10	32/10	33/10

*You'll need to decrease fruit and grain portions to meet 4 grams carbohydrate per kilogram body weight for days 7–5 before competition (see chapter 3).

**You can increase the proportion of calories from fat and decrease the amount from protein by increasing the servings of fat on your program and decreasing the servings of protein/meat substitutes and milk/milk substitutes and still meet your calorie needs.

▶ Peak Performance Carbo-Loading Phase Menus ◀

	DAY 1	**DAY 2**
Morning	Training session—long. Gatorade and Mountain Bar for workout	40 minutes
	Lisa's Scrambled Whites and Greens with Alvarado whole wheat tortillas	Ruth's PR Porridge, fresh fruit
Snack	Fresh fruit smoothie	You Are What You Eat Bar
Afternoon	Lisa's Field of Greens with fat-free Soya Kaas cheese, croutons, and whole grain bread	Abate's Deca-Minestrone, Boboli Bread Sticks
Snack	Balanced Shake	fruits/frozen yogurt, Stretch Island Fruit Leathers
Evening	Ruth's Ironwoman Pho, brown rice, fresh whole-grain bread	Stephens' No Horsing Around Veggie Plate, organic green salad
Snack	Brown's Curling Key Lime Pie	popcorn, Dole fruit pop

	DAY 3	**DAY 4**
Morning	40 minutes	20 minutes
	PowerBar's Protein Plus Bar	Brown's Curling Pre-Meet Combo
Snack	trail mix, apple	mochi w/green tea
Afternoon	Gary's grilled soy cheese on whole wheat, Barbara's oatmeal raisin mini-cookies	Lisa's green salad w/miso dressing, rice crackers
Snack	Hanners' Hummus w/toasted pita	Complete Shake
Evening	Hanners' Red Rice and Beans, steamed carrots	Brown's Curling Kenyan Tortilla, tossed salad
Snack	Häagen-Dazs Sorbet—Mandarin Orange	Luppy's dairy-free pudding snack

	DAY 5	**DAY 6**
Morning	20 minutes	no training—rest
	Charlene's Skating Supplement w/oats, fresh fruit	Met-Rx Bar, water
Snack	Clif Bar, pear	Gatorade/water, high-carb drink
Afternoon	fruit salad, White Wave non-dairy yogurt	veggie sub, banana
Snack	Dave Scott's Pre-Sport Shake	Shiloh Farms spelt or oat bran pretzels

	DAY 5 (CONTINUED)		**DAY 6 (CONTINUED)**
Evening	Didonato's Swimming Rice Primavera, organic tomato and cucumber salad		Wurzel and Mathews' Marathon Pre-Race Pasta Blaster with Gimme Lean meatless balls, small salad
Snack	Tofutti Pop		Hain's Rice Cake—Strawberry Flavor

	DAY 7
Morning	race day
	guarana-rich drink, iced tea, PowerBar
Snack	Campbell's or Ben's pre-meet breakfast meal
Afternoon	After-meet drinks, bagels, fruit pops; take postrace supplements, protein shake, fruit, sport drinks
Snack	
Evening	Slam Dunk Fish Dish, vegetables, salad
Snack	Green tea ice cream

Note: Drink with plenty of water, sport drinks, and green tea. Adapt your personal Nutrition Rx and recommended food servings to the recommended meals above.

Recovery Eating

After the big event is over, it's time to repair and prepare for the next phase of your training regimen. Protein needs may be increased up to 72 hours after long-distance events. Glycogen stores need to be replenished for the next competition. Recovery meals help you replace all energy needs after heavy training or even during times of new training challenges. Several of the VSNG athletes' recipes and favorite snack choices are ideal to include for recovery eating.

On the Road

The biggest challenge the VSNG plant-based athlete faces is finding enough high-quality protein sources and vegetarian foods on the road. In fact, over one-quarter of the VSNG athletes converted from strict vegans to semivegetarians because of this.

▼

Lisa's Field of Greens with Soy Cheese

Makes 1 serving

———

2 cups greens (lettuce, chicory, dandelion,
and other green leafy vegetables)
¼ cup mung bean sprouts, alfalfa sprouts, lentil sprouts
3 oz cubed fat-free Soya Kaas cheese
1 tsp toasted sesame seeds

———

Toss with fat-free dressing or other natural dressing like miso (don't forget to add additional calories, fat, etc., if necessary).

▶ Nutrients per serving: 291 calories, 33 grams protein, 33 grams carbohydrates, 5 grams fat

▶ Dietary composition: 42% protein, 43% carbohydrates, 15% fat

▶ VSNG food servings: ½ grain, 1½ protein, 2½ cups vegetables

▶ Good sources of vitamin A, C, K, folate, potassium, iron; moderate source of B_6, pantothenic acid, calcium, phosphorus, magnesium, copper, manganese

Air Travel

During air travel, the pressurization of the cabin increases fluid losses. These fluid losses may contribute to jet lag. During the flight it is best to have bottled water with you to drink continuously throughout the flight.

Since the airlines are also cutting back on meal service, you may not find your favorite vegetarian meal waiting for you. However, if you do want a special meal, you'll need to call 24 hours in advance to get your request. Some airlines have two vegetarian choices, with dairy or vegetables only. Be sure to ask if they have this option.

If no meal service is planned, bring a variety of snacks on board. My favorite on-board snacks are sport bars, 8-Mate assorted rice cracker snacks with dried peas, Ana Hana brand snack bean party mix, Shiloh Farms oat bran pretzels, Alvarado Street organic whole wheat tortillas, and fresh fruit. I've even been known to pack vegetable sushi for longer lunch and dinner flights. Many airports also have a variety of baked pretzels, frozen yogurt, trail mixes, baked chips, and bagels to purchase at newsstands and snack bars.

The same types of snacks and fluids also can be taken on car or bus trips.

Hotels and Abroad

Erica said the best thing she learned by eating vegetarian is to plan ahead. Jane takes protein shakes and PR Bars on the road. By personal experience, Gary Gromet and his wife prepared days worth of fresh German bread and vegetarian stew prior to the 100th Boston Marathon (sharing this with them may have bought me my 2:53 time!).

The best way to pack plant-based foods for the road is to bring products familiar to you. The next best way is to bring products that can be reconstituted, such as Fantastic Food soups, dips, and dishes, Red Mill's Hot Cereals, Barbara's mashed potatoes, and others listed on the foundation food lists. All you need to add is boiling bottled water!

Be sure to stash plenty of sport bars and powdered carbohydrate replacement fuels, Greens Today, and E-mergen-C packets, and your favorite supplement.

Sometimes you can even get lucky and fly into a city with a fast food restaurant that caters to vegetarian athletes. One of my favorites is Subway for their vegetarian sub, and also Wendy's for their baked potato and salad bar. Other restaurants and their potential plant-based choices are described in the table on the following page.

At hotels, room service often offers a choice of pasta dishes, potatoes, rice, salads, and vegetables. Be sure to ask for a basket of bread plain and crackers and a pitcher of water to wash down and hydrate with your high-carb plant-based meal.

▶ Fast Food and Other Restaurants Offering ◀ Plant-Based Food Choices*

RESTAURANT	FOOD CHOICES
Applebee's	Vegetable Skillet Dish, salads
Arby's	garden salad
Au Bon Pain	bagels, vegetarian soups, salads
Auntie Anne's	hand-rolled pretzels
Baskin-Robbins	ices, sorbets, yogurts
Bojangle's	coleslaw, Cajun pinto beans, corn on the cob, salads
Bonanza	salad bar
Boston Market	steamed veggies, fruit salad, apple cinnamon pie
Bruegger's Bagel Bakery	bagels, soups
Burger King	fries, hash browns, onion rings, French toast sticks, bagels
Chi-Chi's	refried beans, chips and salsa, vegetarian Chajita, dinner salad, guacamole
Chili's	salads, steamed vegetables, tortilla with beans
Chuck E. Cheese	pizza, salads
Church's Fried Chicken	corn on the cob, apple turnover
Country Kitchen International	salads, vegetables, juices
Denny's	cereal combo, bagels, fresh fruit, hot cereal, salad, baked potatoes, spaghetti
Domino's	pizza, salad
El Pollo Loco	spinach and tomato flavored tortillas, pinto beans, corn on the cob, cucumber salad, guacamole, Spanish rice, fiesta corn
Fuddruckers	Vegetarian Fuddwrapper
Howard Johnson	Wholesome and Hearty's Gardenburger, spaghetti, salads
KFC	corn on the cob, garden salad
Long John Silver	The Wrap (order without fish, chicken, or shrimp)
Manchu Wok	stir-fry, rice
McDonald's	garden salad, baked apple pie
Nathan's	Best French fries, made from fresh potatoes and cooked in unused corn oil

continued

▶ *Fast Food and Other Restaurants Offering Plant-Based Food Choices*
(continued)

Pizza Hut	pizza, salad bar
Popeye's	corn on the cob, apple pie
Subway	vegetarian sub on whole wheat, Wholesome and Hearty Gardenburger, White Wave soy turkey subs at certain locations
Taco Bell	corn tortillas, wheat tortillas, pinto beans, chips and salsa, cinnamon twists, Border Ice products
TCBY	frozen yogurt
Wendy's (given high marks by VRG [Vegetarian Resource Group]— See 1/98 issue)	Garden Veggie Pita, salads, baked potato, Mexican Bar

*Adapted from information from the Vegetarian Resource Group, *Vegetarian Journal,* 1/98.

Supermarket Sophistication

Besides an entire newsletter devoted to this topic, being *Supermarket Savvy* (see Appendix C for ordering information) means being wise about your plant-based food choices to get the biggest bang for the buck! Many new terms associated with your favorite foods have suddenly appeared in the aisles. Since they are often trendy and ambiguous, this section will help define the labels you see on your shelves.

Neutraceuticals, a.k.a. Functional Foods

An apple a day keeps the doctor away. Have some chicken soup when you're feeling under the weather. These are a taste of things to come in the year 2000 and beyond—the development of foods for specific purposes.

In 1989 an endocrinologist, Dr. Stephen DeFelice, coined the term *neutraceutical,* defining it as any substance considered a food or part of a food with medical or health benefits, including the prevention, treatment, or cure of disease. Dr. Elizabeth Stone of Applied

Biometrics added that neutraceuticals are foods or beverages that confer health benefits by the addition of ingredients or elimination of unhealthy substances.

Three categories of these foods are:

Lifestyle Foods: Designed to make you feel, look, or perform better. Most sport foods fall into this category.

Disease Prevention Foods: Products added to foods to help prevent the risk of disease. Fiber, antioxidants, and phytochemicals are included here.

Special Needs Foods: Products that help individuals with chronic conditions. Sugar-free snacks for diabetics or fat-free foods for heart patients are examples from this group.

Neutroceuticals have made our lives easier. They have taken some of the thinking out of selecting the best food choices for sport, health, and life. These products often eliminate the need and expense for purchasing excessive vitamin and mineral supplements, or combine the basic nutrition requirements and the desired neutraceutical ingredient of the active or less healthy individual into a drink, shake, or cereal.

Unfortunately, this field is not well regulated. Wiser companies have opted to market their products as supplements instead of as foods, since then they do not come under FDA regulations. Hence, health claims can span a much broader spectrum than if the products were evaluated by the FDA even when not validated by scientific truth. My suggestion is to look carefully at products, try to get most of your nutrients through traditional fresh and wholesome food sources, and rely on neutraceuticals for special times like Jane does on the road to racing—she uses drinks and bars only when competing.

Organically Grown

Do you feel like you're buying something healthier and better for the environment when you purchase organically grown food? You should. After all, you and other health-conscious, fitness-minded individuals are spending $4 billion a year for that very reason.

In 1990, Congress passed the Organic Foods Production Act, which calls for the establishment of national organic guidelines.

These guidelines include certification for growers, screening of organic imports, monitoring of chemical contamination, evaluation of livestock living conditions, and development of standards for production. The National Organic Standards Board (NOSB) consists of farmers, food processors, retailers, scientists, environmentalists, and consumer advocates to assist the United States Department of Agriculture (USDA) in developing standards. Right now only eleven states require that crops and foods be certified organic, and each state has slightly different terminology.

What is organic? The criterion for organic products is to have 95 % organically produced ingredients, excluding water and salt. Products with 50 to 95% organic ingredients can only use the phrase "made with certain organic ingredients."

Despite the positive support of the government toward regulating chemical-free food, there have been several oversights in the program. These oversights include the irradiation of foods to kill disease-causing bacteria; fertilization of crops with sewage sludge, called biosolids; and genetically engineered foods to resist pests. Since you can be assured that some of the states have strong programs, I recommend that you continue to purchase certain organic products such as fruit, vegetables, and canned goods over nonorganic versions. One of the best ways to be assured of your food's "organic-ness" is to purchase your foods through a Community Supported Agricultural (CSA) system.

Community-Supported Agriculture (CSA)

A CSA system is a partnership between local farmers and consumers. In exchange for financial support from consumers in the form of a membership, farmers provide a share of the annual harvest. The first CSA programs were started in Japan about 30 years ago and began in this country in 1986. Today more than 600 CSA systems operate across the United States and Canada. Since most food eaten travels 1,300 miles from farmer to dinner table, CSA programs save on fossil fuels that contribute to global warming; ensure fresh food, often picked the morning of delivery; and offer consumers organically grown choices.

About 1,000 farms have been lost annually in the last decade. As farms disappear, so does the special relationship between the growers and the community. CSA is a cost-effective way to save those farms and feed plant-based, fitness-minded individuals an exciting array of fresh food.

Typically, consumers pay the farmer before the season starts, in order to cover operating costs. The CSA membership is based on shares of the harvest. In one CSA program in New York, a share price of $263 brings 30 weeks of 10 pounds of seasonally selected, organically grown vegetables delivered at a cost of less than a dollar per pound. To keep the fees low, members volunteer about 3 hours per season for every share they buy. They donate their time by working in the office, doing paperwork, or unloading trucks.

Joining a CSA program is an easy way to get a greater variety of plant-based foods, provide an element of surprise at mealtime, and bring back a community spirit that so many are missing these days. To find out more about CSA in your community, call your local farmers' market or cooperative extension service. Other resources include:

Bio Dynamic Farming and Gardens Association
List of CSAs in North America
800-516-7797

Environmental Nutrition Dietetic Practice Group
    of the American Dietetic Association
800-877-1600, ext. 4815
Web site: HYPERLINK http://www.eatright.org/dpg

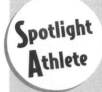

Spotlight Athlete

Erika Brown

1998 Olympic curler
All Big Ten MVP Golfer

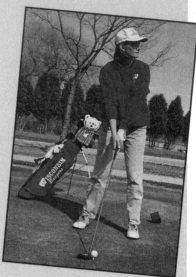

Age: 25

8 years lacto-ovo-vegetarian

Reason for becoming vegetarian:
"I eliminated meat from my diet for both health and ethical reasons. I think it is possible to be a healthy, active, energized athlete without eating meat and contributing to the subsequent environmental damage that accompanies its production."

Advantages of being vegetarian:
"It's quite a rarity. People take notice when they find out and with any luck take a closer look at their own diet."

Challenges to being vegetarian: "Many curling tournaments are held in small Midwestern towns of the strictly meat-and-potatoes variety. Often, meals are served right at the curling facility, which further decreases my options for food. It's been a good lesson in planning ahead."

Alcohol: occasionally beer or wine

Supplements: none

Favorite precompetition meal: Brown's Curling Pre-Meet Combo (page 214)

Favorite snacks: fruit, fruit shakes (made with low-fat yogurt or ice cream), pretzels, trail mix

Favorite one-pot meals: Brown's Curling Kenyan Tortilla (page 103) and Brown's Curling Key Lime Pie (page 229)

Debbie Stephens

World-class equestrian show jumper

Age: 47

18 years pesco-vegetarian

Reason for becoming vegetarian: "Wanted to lose weight, have more energy, and be more energetic."

Advantages of being vegetarian: "More energy, feel healthier."

Challenges to being vegetarian: "Hard to get food to eat at competition sites."

Alcohol: none

Supplements: none

Favorite premeet meal: Stephens' No Horsing Around Precompetition Snack (page 213), candy bar, and coffee (see chapter 6 for a summary on the benefits of caffeine)

Favorite snacks: candy

Favorite one-pot meal: Stephens' No Horsing Around Veggie Plate (page 150)

Hanners' Apple Tower Dessert

Makes 4 servings

———

3 firm, ripe apples, Braeburn or Macintosh

$\frac{1}{2}$ cup dried cranberries

$\frac{1}{2}$ cup oats, whole

$\frac{1}{4}$ cup brown sugar

$\frac{1}{4}$ cup flour

1 tbs soft soy margarine

1 lemon zest

1 tsp cinnamon

1 tsp nutmeg

1 tsp clove

———

Peel and core apples. Slice apples paper-thin and make 4 stacks, using $\frac{3}{4}$ apple for each stack. In a small bowl, combine all remaining ingredients. Stuff apples with mixture. Bake uncovered at 350°F for 50 minutes.

Apple Caramel Drizzle

$\frac{3}{4}$ cup sugar

2 tbs water

$\frac{1}{2}$ cup apple juice

———

Bring sugar and water to caramel stage. When amber in color, add apple juice carefully and whisk rapidly. Drizzle over apple tower.

▶ Nutrients per serving: 402 calories, 4 grams protein, 90 grams carbohydrates, 5 grams fat, 1 gram monounsaturated fat, 1.5 grams linoleic fat, 64 grams sugar, 5 grams fiber

▶ Dietary composition: 4% protein, 85% carbohydrates, 11% fat

▶ VSNG food servings: 1$\frac{1}{2}$ fruits, 1$\frac{1}{2}$ grains, 1 fat

▶ Source of manganese

Brown's Curling Key Lime Pie

Makes 8 servings

————

ready-to-bake piecrust

8 oz fresh or bottled lime juice

1 can sweetened condensed milk

4 cups fat-free or low-fat vanilla ice cream

————

Blend lime juice, sweetened condensed milk, and ice cream. Pour into piecrust. Let chill in freezer for at least 2 hours.

▶ Nutrients per serving: 206 calories, 5 grams protein, 36 grams carbohydrates, 5 grams fat, 1 gram saturated fat, 55 mg sodium

▶ Dietary composition: 10% protein, 70% carbohydrates, 20% fat

▶ VSNG food servings: 1/2 milk, 1 1/2 grains, and 1 fat

▶ No major source of any vitamins or minerals

Vegetarian Athletes' Nutritional Profiles

Warmup

This section provides you with the spotlight athletes' typical one-day food diaries and a nutritional analysis (analyzed by using the Nutritionist IV software program). In no way can one day reflect an entire dietary intake, but it can give you an idea of the relationship between a specific food intake and the nutrients you find in those foods. In scientific research, three-to-seven-day food diaries are often kept to establish a pattern of eating.

Since this was not scientific research, to respect the athletes' valuable voluntary time, I asked and was grateful to get at least a typical 24-hour period. Some athletes had to e-mail or send the diaries to me from all parts of the world, some while competing. Some included foods, bars, drinks, and snacks that were manually added to the computer analysis program. Therefore, some of the vitamin and mineral data may not be complete.

Remember also that some of these athletes, such as Dave, Art, Jonathon, and Chris, have retired from their sports and no longer consume their training diets. Their intakes reflect the diets they are presently consuming.

In the Food Fitness section, I did not try to change everything about the athletes' dietary intake. The purpose of the Food Fitness section is to show you how a vegetarian sports nutritionist and athlete may slightly adjust their present diets to satisfied their personal eating needs and improve their profiles to better meet their dietary goals. Obviously, these habits, healthy or not, have helped these athletes to achieve some of the highest goals in their sports. Also, as a licensed psychotherapist, I am careful not to change everything about the person, since dramatic changes often do not last.

Benefiting from These Nutritional Profiles

These twenty-four-hour intakes can demonstrate how an athlete from your favorite sport can sustain strength and endurance on plant-based diets. You can use these profiles to compare your typical daily intake to theirs. By using this information, you can improve the nutritional quality of your diet by helping you select foods and nutrients to complement your present diet. It may also help you to choose an appropriate nutritional supplement when food can't meet your needs. Additional information on supplementation is found in chapter 8.

Your Personal Nutritionist

If you are serious about your food and sport, you may choose to continue working with a sports nutritionist, online or in person.

If you would like to work with me personally, just send the Food Fitness Nutritional Analysis and Activity form from Appendix B by fax, mail, or e-mail to me at the addresses provided. I will send you back a personal Nutritional Prescription (Rx) and nutrition and training program and menus. You can even have your favorite recipes analyzed and included in your daily diet.

If you prefer to work with someone in person, in your hometown or abroad, you can contact one of the groups listed in Appendix C to give you a list of referrals in the city you desire.

If you have any other questions, concerns, or comments, log onto my Web site (www.lisadorfman.com).

▶ Section 1: Spotlight ◀ Semivegetarian Athletes

Jonathan Didonato

Guinness Book of Records swimmer
Spotlight athlete, chapter 5

One-day food diary

Meal one	two oranges, one grapefruit
Meal two	one banana, one apple
Meal three	one apple, one banana
Meal four	Power Shake, Rx Fuel with egg whites
Meal five	salad
Meal six	Power Shake
Meal seven	Didonato's Swimming Rice Primavera (see page 104)
Supplements	spirulina and bee pollen

Dietary composition

17% protein, 73% carbohydrates, 10% fat

Nutritional analysis without supplements

Calories: 2,394
Carbohydrates: 460 grams
Protein: 105 grams
Fat: 27 grams
Saturated fat: 5 grams
Cholesterol: 2 milligrams
Sugar: 201 grams (50 tsp)
Fiber: 65 grams
Vitamins and minerals
   All except vitamin D are between 70% and 1,457% RDAs.
   Deficiencies: vitamin D, 0% RDA

Food fitness suggestions: Reduce sugar intake by selecting less fruits and by substituting one low-sugar sport shake daily. Since Jonathan lives and works in the south Florida sun, he is getting vitamin D. His sport shakes are also fortified with vitamins and minerals. He can also include a fortified milk-based, soy or rice milk daily.

Ben Richardson

Laser sailor
Spotlight athlete, chapter 6

One-day food diary

7:00 A.M.	32 oz water
8:00 A.M.	2 cups oatmeal w/ soy milk and soy protein, 24 grams
12:30 P.M.	salad and tofu (alternates)
3:30 P.M.	Balance Bar
6:30 P.M.	dinner w/ fish or chicken
Extras	beer, ice cream
Supplements	chromium, creatine

Dietary composition
35% protein, 43% carbohydrates, 22% fat

Nutritional analysis without supplements
Calories: 1,654
Carbohydrates: 185 grams
Protein: 153 grams
Fat: 42 grams
Saturated Fat: 4 grams
Cholesterol: 172 milligrams
Sugar: 17 grams (4 tsp)
Fiber: 13 grams
Vitamins and minerals
  All except vitamin D and biotin, between 65% and 727% RDAs
  Deficiencies: vitamin D, 0% RDA, biotin; 28% RDA

Food fitness suggestions: Consume a greater proportion of carbohydrate-rich food for energy (it probably increases with the ice cream and beer!) Additional fruits and vegetables would improve carbohydrate and fiber intake. Balance Bar and others are also fortified with D and biotin.

Art Still

Football player
Spotlight athlete, chapter 4

One-day food diary

6:00 A.M.   1 quart of water, green tea, and fresh-squeezed lemon

6:15 A.M.   workout

7:30–8:00 A.M. 3 pancakes, 6 egg whites

10–10:30 A.M.   fruit (bananas, apple, or fruit shake with banana, frozen strawberries, and orange juice)

12:00 P.M.   turkey sandwich or a couple of Boca Burgers w/cheese sandwich

3:00 P.M.   fruit

5:30 P.M.   stir-fry or beans and rice (see Still's "Defensive" Stir-Fry recipe on page 82)

Supplements   Nutri Rx w/ creatine, multivitamin

Dietary composition
22% protein, 69% carbohydrates, 9% fat

Nutritional analysis without supplements
Calories: 1,880
Carbohydrates: 330 grams
Protein: 104 grams
Fat: 19 grams
Saturated fat: 5 grams
Cholesterol: 157 milligrams
Sugar: 124 grams (31 tsp)
Fiber: 38 grams
Vitamins and minerals
    All vitamins and minerals are between 55% and 435% RDAs except vitamins D, E, K, and A and biotin.
    Deficiencies: vitamin D, 0% RDA; vitamin K, 5% RDA

Food fitness suggestions: The vitamins found to be deficient in Art's diet are probably included in his supplement. Because Art lives in the north, vitamin D needs to come through food sources, as he can't rely on sunlight as a source (see chapter 7). A and K can be included in additional servings of deep green vegetables. Vitamin D can be found in fortified soy or rice milk and/or sport shakes.

Debbie Stephens

World-class equestrian show jumper
Spotlight athlete, chapter 10

One-day food diary

7:00 A.M.	1 bagel, 4 cups coffee
Lunch	salad, 3 Diet Cokes
3:00 P.M.	cookies, chocolate bar, coffee
8:00 P.M.	salad, fish, Stephens' No Horsing Around Veggie Plate (see page 150)
	Diet Coke
Supplements	none

Dietary composition

34% protein, 55% carbohydrates, 11% fat

Nutritional analysis without supplements

Calories: 1,128
Carbohydrates: 159 grams
Protein: 99 grams
Fat: 14 grams
Saturated fat: 2 grams
Cholesterol: 215 milligrams
Sugar: 36 grams (9 tsp)
Fiber: 30 grams
Vitamins and minerals
   All are between 50% and 868% RDAs except biotin, vitamins D and
      E, and calcium.
   Deficiencies: vitamin D, 0% RDAs; caffeine intake

Food fitness suggestions: Although the calories are low for sport, the percentages from protein, carbohydrates, and fats help Debbie manage her weight and energy levels for world-class competition. The high protein intake probably helps to manage her blood sugar levels and appetite between meals. However, this high-protein, extremely low-fat diet may cause her to crave sugars and cause calcium losses from bone.

   Realizing that Debbie likes sweets and chocolate, I would suggest a daily chocolate sport bar to replace the candy bar and some of the caffeine from the Diet Cokes she consumes daily. Perhaps one espresso with milk (or fortified soy milk) in the morning instead of 4 cups coffee would provide the caffeine "fix" and give her a bit more calcium and D. There are also many natural teas that can provide Debbie with a natural kick (see New Age fluids in chapter 6) and a better replacement of liquids.

Dina Head

WNBA player
Spotlight athlete, chapter 9

One-day food diary

9:30 A.M.	24 oz protein shake
12:30 P.M.	16 oz ice tea, medium salad plate w/ tomatoes, cucumbers, salmon
Snack	fruit, graham crackers, or handful of nuts
4:00 P.M.	16 oz water
7:00 P.M.	8 oz steamed vegetables
10:00 P.M.	Head's Slam Dunk Fish Dish (see page 102)
Supplements	vitamins E, C, B_{12}, and multivitamin

Dietary composition
26% protein, 60% carbohydrates, 14% fat

Nutritional analysis without supplements
Calories: 1,675
Carbohydrates: 250 grams
Protein: 109 grams
Fat: 26 grams
Saturated fat: 3 grams
Cholesterol: 157 milligrams
Sugar: 83 grams (20 tsp)
Fiber: 32 grams
Vitamins and minerals
   All are between 67% and 703% RDAs.

Food fitness suggestions: Beautiful dietary composition, great sources of vitamins and minerals. Good job, Dina!

Gary Gromet

Ironman triathlete and marathon runner
Spotlight athlete, chapter 5

One-day food diary

1 1/2 Parillo Bars

4.5 liters water

1 scoop Ripped fuel

3 servings Cytomax, 56 oz fluid

10 slices multigrain bread

5 1/2 servings Kamut puffed cereal

64 grams whey protein powder

1/2 cup raisins

rolled oats—1 cup dry

tofu, baked—4 oz

tofu cheese—2 oz

1 red pepper

1 yellow pepper

1 cup sauerkraut

2/3 cup dry roasted soybeans

1 pumpernickel bagel

2 cups salad

1 cup spinach

1/2 lb salmon

1 1/2 cups rice

1 frozen fruit and protein treat

1 glass red wine

12 oz nonalcoholic beer

Supplements: vitamins C and E, magnesium, creatine, carnitine, ginkgo biloba, pycnogenal, grapeseed, phosphatidyl serine, melatonin, alpha lipoic acid, glucosamine, glutamine, gluthathionine, ginseng, HMG, ferrochal bisglycinate, lycopene, CoQ10, beta carotene, phytoflavinoids, tribulus, tennestris

Dietary composition

22% protein, 58% carbohydrates, 17% fat

Nutritional analysis without supplements

Calories: 4,237

Carbohydrates: 654 grams

Protein: 248 grams

Fat: 83 grams

Saturated fat: 10 grams

Cholesterol: 111 milligrams

Sugar: 51 grams (12 tsp)

Fiber: 37 grams

Vitamins and minerals

   All are between 59% and 512% RDAs.

   Deficiencies: vitamin D, 0% RDA; biotin, 44% RDA

Food fitness suggestions: It's amazing that Gary gets all the nutrients in such great percentages except, like the other athletes, D and biotin. Gary has no problem getting D from the hot south Florida sunshine. He takes so many supplements, but being in the health food business, it's hard for him to resist the temptations of new and exciting research. I've known Gary for more than 10 years, and I can tell you firsthand that he is an amazing man, with no health problems and the body of a twenty-year-old. Perhaps his present diet and supplement program enables him to perform for more than four hours daily in training.

Dave Scott

Six-time ironman champion
Spotlight athlete, chapter 8

One-day food diary

Breakfast	Dave Scott's Pre-Sport Shake (see page 128)
	2 scoops Metabol II (240 calories, 24 grams protein, 10 grams fat, 13.5 grams carbohydrates),
	2 pieces whole wheat toast
	1 PowerBar
Midmorning	2 apples
	1 PowerBar
Lunch	bagel sandwich—lettuce, tomato, onion, sprouts, and hummus spread (see Hanners' Hummus, page 24)
	second bagel
	2 apples
	Odwalla super protein shake
Midday	PowerBar and bagel
Dinner	1 can tuna
	2 cups dry pasta
	olive oil
	large salad
	1/2 bag bean chips
	1 bowl frozen nonfat yogurt
	6–8 Fig Newtons
Supplements	vitamins E and C, iron, and beta carotene

Dietary composition
19% protein, 65% carbohydrates, 16% fat

Nutritional analysis without supplements
Calories: 5,028
Carbohydrates: 850 grams
Protein: 249 grams
Fat: 95 grams
Saturated fat: 14 grams
Cholesterol: 87 milligrams
Sugar: 226 grams (56 tsp)
Fiber: 54 grams
Vitamins and minerals
    All except vitamin D are between 75% and 651% RDAs.

Food fitness suggestions: Since Dave lives in Colorado, he may get sunshine to convert to vitamin D; through food, he may be able to get more D with a cup or two of D-fortified soy drink or yogurt. His sport bar is also fortified with vitamin D; however, since his sugar intake is so high, he might want to have a lower-sugar bar or drink instead.

▶ Section 2: Spotlight ◀ Lacto-Ovo-Vegetarian Athletes

Jane Welzel

1990 U.S. national marathon champion, 2:33 marathoner
Spotlight athlete, chapter 3

One-day food diary

8:00 A.M.	mocha espresso with skim milk and chocolate
12:30 P.M.	tofu cheese sandwich on whole wheat with lettuce, mustard, and seitan
3:00 P.M.	crackers and tofu cheese
6:30 P.M.	seitan, rice, vegetables, and a glass of wine
8:00 P.M.	jelly beans
Supplements	vitamin C, iron, multivitamin (PR Bar and protein powder when away from home)

Dietary composition

18% protein, 62% carbohydrates, 15% fat

Nutritional analysis without supplements

Calories: 1,239

Carbohydrates: 212 grams

Protein: 62 grams

Fat: 22 grams

Saturated fat: 3 grams

Cholesterol: 4 milligrams

Sugar: 49 (12.25 tsp)

Fiber: 15 grams

Vitamins and minerals

Good sources of vitamins A, B_1, B_2, B_3, B_6, B_{12}, and K, folate, potassium, calcium, phosphorus, magnesium, iron, zinc, copper, manganese, and selenium.

Food fitness suggestions: Jane's snacks of tofu pops, popcorn, candy, tortilla chips, crackers, and hummus probably add additional calories needed to support her training but are not accounted for in this assessment. She may benefit from a daily fortified sports bar to ensure meeting calorie and vitamin and mineral needs and a daily serving of a VSNG spotlight athlete's recipe chock full of nutrients and fiber like Ruth's Ironwoman Pho.

Erika Brown

Olympic curler and All-American golfer
Spotlight athlete, chapter 10

One-day food diary

8:00 A.M.   1 glass orange juice, 1 bowl cereal—$^1/_2$ Cheerios, $^1/_2$ Grape Nuts, and skim milk

1:00 P.M.   1 banana, skim milk, vegetable soup, 2 slices whole wheat toast

6:00 P.M.   skim milk and vegetable stir-fry with rice (see Still's "Defensive" Stir-Fry on page 82)

Supplements   none

Dietary composition

16% protein, 75% carbohydrates, 9% fat

Nutritional analysis without supplements
Calories: 1,700
Carbohydrates: 332 grams
Protein: 73 grams
Fat: 17 grams
Saturated fat: 3 grams
Cholesterol: 12 milligrams
Sugar: 104 grams (26 tsp)
Fiber: 33 grams
Vitamins and minerals
All are between 94% and 821% RDAs except biotin (49%) and
vitamin E (37%).

Food fitness suggestions: Erika is an excellent eater and probably gets
even more calories, fat, and vitamin E with her trail mix, fruit, fruit
shake, and/or pretzel snacks. Ruth's Ironwoman Pho would ensure her
E intake. No need for supplements here!

Lisa Dorfman

Author, triathlete, and distance runner

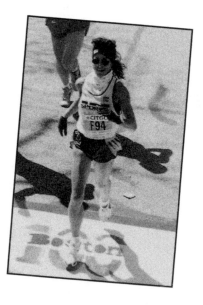

Typical one-day food diary
Every day
    1–2 liters Evian water, sport drinks,
    8–16 oz caffeinated drink—tea,
    1–2 sport bars, Starbucks Coffee
    Frappuccino, fresh fruit smoothies,
    natural sorbets, frozen soy desserts,
    or frozen fruit pops and/or sport
    shake
Before training 5:00 A.M.
    caffeinated tea or other drink,
    about 50 mg and water
During and after morning workout
    sport bar, Gatorade, Cytomax, or XLR8 sport drink, supplements
Midmorning: 2–3 times per week
    Starbucks Coffee Frappuccino; fruit, organic whole wheat tor-
    tillas, 8-grain rolls

About 10:30–11:00 A.M.

Lisa's Scrambled Whites and Greens (see page 77), soy cheese and apple, or poppyseed cracker flats, cheese flatbreads, dried fruits (strawberries, blueberries, bananas, figs rolled in coconut, plain figs, raisins, apricots, and/or peaches), frozen fruit pops

12:00–1:30 P.M.

Lisa's Field of Greens with Soy Cheese and miso dressing, croutons, and/or crackers; whole wheat tortilla or 8-grain roll

3:00–6:00 P.M.

snacks consisting of either or a combination of dried peas, dried fruits, frozen yogurt, crackerbread, pasta chips, flour or corn tortillas, Fantastic Foods Bean or Hummus Dip with tortillas or Baked Lays Chips, fresh fruit, or fruit smoothie

Dinner (always a minimum of 2 to 3 hours before bedtime)

whole wheat or Quinoa pasta, risotto, couscous, quinoa, or rice with peas, corn, and broccoli, or baked or mashed potatoes with greens, tamales, baked taco pie and/or plain tomato, spinach or whole wheat tortillas

Evening sweet snack

depends on many factors: frozen sorbet or yogurt, Arrowhead Mills Coco O's with fortified soy drink, Tofutti Chocolate Fudge Treat, or natural organic licorice

Supplements

Almost daily—Alacer Super Gram multivitamin, Twinlab's Antioxidant Fuel or Oxy Quencher; with heavy training, racing, and/or intermittently depending on diet and needs—Twinlab's Phos Fuel, Anti-Catabolic Fuel, Lipotropic Fuel, Carni Fuel, Slow Fe with Folic Acid, and/or E-Mergen-C

Dietary composition
21% protein, 69% carbohydrates, 10% fat

Nutritional analysis without supplements, sport drinks, or shakes
Calories: 2,112
Carbohydrates: 371 grams
Protein: 114 grams
Fat: 25 grams
Saturated fat: 4 grams
Cholesterol: 42 milligrams

Sugar: 84 grams (21 tsp)

Fiber: 28 grams

Vitamins and minerals

Good sources of vitamins A, B_1, B_2, B_3, B_6, C, K, folate, pantothenic acid, potassium, calcium, phosphorus, magnesium, iron, zinc, copper, and manganese—between 54% (zinc) and 938% (K) RDAs

Moderate to minimal sources of vitamins B_{12}, D (0%), E, biotin, selenium

Food fitness suggestions: Between my sport bar, shakes, vitamin and mineral supplements (not included in the analysis), and the south Florida sun, I have no concern about getting enough vitamin D and minerals found in short supply, although I vary my diet throughout the year, and my supplements change according to training (marathon vs. short distance), climate (winter vs. summer oppression), and my monthly menstrual cycle.

At 5'3" and 104 pounds (47 kilograms), I eat approximately 45 calories per kilogram, 2.4 grams of protein per kilogram (much higher during the present marathon training than other times of the year), and 8 grams of carbohydrates per kilogram, which perfectly meets my needs. I never seem to have recovery problems or get dehydrated except at the inception of the summer season in south Florida, when the temperatures and humidity go from 70° and 70 to 80% humidity to 85 to 100° and 90 to 100% humidity overnight!

I train half the amount of time as my counterparts, averaging 1 to 2 hours daily of running (40–60 miles per week), swimming (3,000–9,000 yards per week), cycling, and weights.

I feel and look younger than 38 (so I'm told), have had three healthy pregnancies and deliveries, bouncing back to training and normal weight within weeks while breastfeeding, have a normal menstrual cycle, and have never suffered from anemia since becoming a vegetarian at age fifteen. My body fat was measured for two research studies in 1993 and 1996 and was a lean 11% and 9% respectively. This is my personal testimony to the adequacy and validity of my lacto-ovo plant-based diet.

▶ Section 3: Spotlight ◀ Vegan Athletes

Craig Heath

Professional figure skater
Spotlight athlete, chapter 7

One-day food diary

Daily	1 gallon distilled water
Snacks	peanut butter and jelly, rice cakes, or health nut cookies
Morning	raisin granola, banana, and soymilk
Lunch	vegetarian burrito, refried beans, salsa lettuce, tomato, rice corn, and tofu
Dinner	pasta with tomato sauce, or potato or 3 cups rice, with a side of vegetables

Supplements   Super Nutrition vitamin packs, echinacea, goldenseal, DHEA, glucosamine, sodium chondroitin, two energy drinks: one with caffeine and green tea and the other with arginine

Dietary composition
13% protein, 74% carbohydrates, 13% fat

Nutritional analysis without supplements
Calories: 1,722
Carbohydrates: 328
Protein: 56 grams
Fat: 26 grams
Saturated fat: 10 grams
Cholesterol: 13 milligrams
Sugar: 29 grams (7 tsp)
Fiber: 22 grams
Vitamins and minerals
   Good sources of vitamins A, B_1, B_2, B_3, B_6, folate, pantothenic acid, potassium, phosphorus, magnesium, iron, copper, manganese
   Moderate sources of vitamin B_{12}, C, calcium, zinc
   Deficiencies: low in D, 0% RDA; selenium, 6% RDA

Food fitness suggestions: Craig can benefit from a daily snack of peanut butter and jelly on whole wheat and a glass of vitamin D and B_{12}–fortified soy or rice drink. His energy drinks help him to meet his vitamin/mineral and additional calorie needs.

Ruth Heidrich

Ironwoman and marathon runner
Spotlight athlete, chapter 1

One-day food diary

Morning	1 1/2 cups oatmeal and greens
Midday	Ruth's Ironwoman Pho (Vietnamese soup; see page 149)
3:00 P.M.	3 cups brown rice and vegetables
5:00 P.M.	baked potato, salsa, and carrots
8:00 P.M.	6 cups popcorn, 1 apple
Supplements	none

Dietary composition
16% protein, 78% carbohydrates, 6% fat

Nutritional analysis without supplements
Calories: 1,786
Carbohydrates: 357 grams
Protein: 76 grams
Fat: 12 grams
Saturated fat: 2 grams
Cholesterol: 4 milligrams
Sugar: 57 grams (8 tsp)
Fiber: 52 grams
Vitamins and minerals
　　All are between 75% and 1,222% RDAs except B_{12} and D (0%).

Food fitness suggestions: Since Ruth lives and trains in Hawaii, she probably gets enough D conversion through sunlight; she may benefit from including a glass or two of B_{12} and D–fortified soy or rice milk daily.

Charlene Wong Williams

Olympian and professional figure skater
Spotlight athlete, chapter 6

One-day food diary

Rising	½ cup juice or water with lemon
Breakfast	protein drink, hot cereal, or rice and beans, with tea
Lunch	tempeh and greens or stir-fry with tofu
Snack	vegetable juice or fruit or 8–10 corn chips
Dinner	grain and beans, or tofu green veggies and mixed steamed veggies
Supplements:	Charlene's Skating Supplement (see page 169)

Dietary composition
25% protein, 47% carbohydrates, 28% fat

Nutritional analysis without supplements
Calories: 1,436
Carbohydrates: 179 grams
Protein: 93 grams
Fat: 47 grams
Saturated fat: 5 grams
Cholesterol: 0
Sugar: 27 grams (6¾ tsp)
Fiber: 30 grams
Vitamins and minerals
   All are between 59% and 1,448% RDAs except biotin (9%)
   and D (0%).

Food fitness suggestions: Charlene probably eats slightly more calories than this one-day diary reflects, since she "eats until full" with vegetables, rice, and other grains, although this is difficult to guesstimate within the scope of this analysis. She can benefit from a daily serving of Didonato's Swimming Rice Primavera (page 104) and a vitamin-D-fortified soy or rice drink or a low-sugar, vitamin-enriched sport bar, for additional carbohydrate energy and a vitamin-D-fortified soy or rice drink.

Ben Mathews

Masters marathon sensation
Spotlight athlete, chapter 3

One-day food diary
Daily   bagel for snack
8:00 A.M.   bowl of grape nuts and soymilk, glass of orange juice
1:30 P.M.   rice, beans, and salad
7:00 P.M.   pasta salad and raisins
Supplements   none

Dietary composition
14% protein, 80% carbohydrates, 6% fat

Nutritional analysis without supplements
Calories: 1,857
Carbohydrates: 389 grams
Protein: 68 grams
Fat: 13 grams
Saturated fat: 2 grams
Cholesterol: 28 milligrams
Sugar: 93 grams (23 tsp)
Fiber: 24 grams
Vitamins and minerals
    All between 68% and 613% RDAs except biotin (36%) and calcium
    (40%)

Food fitness suggestions: Ben can benefit from Didonato's Swimming
Rice Primavera (page 104) and a calcium-fortified soy drink or tofu
product. He may also benefit from a macro-based sport bar or drink
fortified with his low intake of biotin and calcium.

Kim Wurzel

U.S. national team synchronized swimmer
Spotlight athlete, chapter 9

One-day food diary

5:30 A.M.	bowl of Corn Flakes or Rice Krispies
10:00 A.M.	PowerBar with Gatorade
2:30 P.M.	hummus sandwich with lemonade
7:30 P.M.	vegetable stir-fry or black bean burritos or baked potato with steamed veggies and small salad
Daily snacks	fruit and saltine crackers
Supplements	creatine powder

Dietary composition
13% protein, 76% carbohydrates, 11% fat

Nutritional analysis without supplements
Calories: 1,254
Carbohydrates: 248 grams
Protein: 44 grams
Fat: 16 grams
Saturated fat: 2 grams
Cholesterol: 5 milligrams
Sugar: 63 grams (about 16 tsp)
Fiber: 24 grams
Vitamins and minerals
    All between 60% and 1,065% RDAs except biotin (27%), D (9%),
    E (49%), and calcium (41%)

Food fitness suggestions: Kim can benefit from additional calories to meet the demands of training for her sport. She can also meet her vitamin and mineral needs from a sport shake or bar, a fortified soy drink, or yogurt as a snack.

Food Fitness Nutritional Activity Assessment Form

Now it's your turn to get analyzed. Here's how easy it is!

List all foods, drinks, condiments, and candy you have consumed during the last three days. It is ideal to use one weekend day and two weekdays (e.g., Sunday, Monday, and Tuesday or Thursday, Friday, and Saturday).

Give the time, food/drink, and amount, as well as a description of the activity you perform during those days. For example:

Food Diary
8:00 A.M.: 1 cup brewed
coffee with 1 % milk, light,
and 1 Sweet and Low

Activity Diary
8:15 A.M.: drop the kids at
school and head to gym
for a 1-hour aerobic class and
$^1/_2$ hour weights.

Date: _____

Food Diary   **Activity Diary**

_____   _____
_____   _____
_____   _____
_____   _____
_____   _____
_____   _____
_____   _____
_____   _____

List all supplements you consume and their dosages. Include specific sport bars, drinks, and gels.

_____
_____
_____

List all medications, including anti-inflammatory drugs and birth control pills, that you take on a daily basis.

_____
_____
_____

List your sport of choice, the amount of time you train per week, and other sports you enjoy on a regular basis.

_____
_____
_____

List any previous or current health problems, concerns, or challenges.

_____
_____
_____

List the primary and secondary reasons for desiring a change in your dietary program.

_____

_____

_____

General Information:

Name _____ Age _____

Address _____

City _____ State _____ Zip _____

Phone_____ fax _____

e-mail_____

Educational level _____

Present occupation _____

Married? _____ Children? _____

How many? _____

Weight _____ Height _____

Weight changes in the last five years? _____

Percent body fat_____

Other pertinent information about your weight distribution:

_____

_____

_____

Favorite foods _____

Least desirable foods _____

Send the Food Fitness Nutrition Activity Assessment form to
Lisa Dorfman, MS, RD, LMHC,
7000 SW 62 Avenue, Suite 350,
Miami, Florida 33143;
or fax to The Running Nutritionist, (305) 662-2854;
or e-mail to foodfitnes@aol.com;
or log onto www.runningnutritionist.com and follow instructions.

Sports and Vegetarian Nutrition Resources

For referrals to qualified sports nutritionists (RDs) who specialize in plant-based diets, contact:

The American Dietetic Association
1-800-877-1600, ext. 4842
www.eatright.org

or contact the Dietetic Practice Group (DPG) of the American Dietetic Association, which can give you more information or a referral to a sports nutritionist who specializes in plant-based diets.

Nutrition Entrepreneurs Dietetic Practice Group (NE)
www.nutritionentrepreneurs.com

Organizations you can join for vegetarian information and networking experiences

Vegetarian Resource Group
P.O. Box 1463
Baltimore, MD 21203
www.vrg.org
410-366-VEGE

North American Vegetarian Society
Box 72
Dolgeville, NY 13329
518-568-7970
navs@telenet.net

Vegetarian magazines

Vegetarian Times
Subscription orders and information: 800-829-3340
www.vegetariantimes.com

Veggie Life
Subscription orders and information: 925-671-9852
www.veggielife.com

Oldways Preservation & Exchange Trust
25 First Street
Cambridge, MA 02141
617-621-3000

Vegetarian Journal
410-366-VEGE
www.vrg.org/journal/address.htm

General health and nutrition newsletters to keep you on the cutting edge of research

Tufts Diet and Nutrition Newsletter
Subscriptions orders and information: 1-800-274-7581
www.healthletter.tufts.edu

Nutrition Action Health Letter
Subscription orders and information:
Center for Science in the Public Interest
1875 Connecticut Avenue NW, Suite 300
Washington, DC 20009-5728
www.cspinet.org

Loma Linda University Vegetarian Nutrition and Health Newsletter
Subscription orders and information: 888-558-8703
vegletter@sph.llu.edu

Supermarket Savvy
Linda McDonald, RD, Editor
Subscription orders and information: 888-577-2889
info@supermarketsavvy.com

The McDougall Newsletter
P.O. Box 14039
Santa Rosa, CA 95402
707-576-1654

Sports nutrition books for your peak-performance library

Applegate, Liz. *Power Foods: High-Performance Nutrition for High-Performance People* (Rodale Press, 1994).

Burke, Edmund, and Berning, Jacqueline. *Training Nutrition* (Cooper Publishing, 1996).

Burke, Louise. *The Complete Guide to Food for Sports Performance*, second edition (Allen and Unwin, 1995).

Clark, Nancy. *Sports Nutrition Guidebook*, second edition (Human Kinetics, 1997).

Coleman, Ellen. *Eating for Endurance* (Bull Publishing, 1988).

Colgan, Michael. *Optimum Sports Nutrition: Your Competitive Edge* (Advanced Research Press, 1993).

Kleiner, Susan, and Greenwood-Robinson, Maggie. *High Performance Nutrition* (John Wiley and Sons, 1996).

Cookbooks

You can call the Vegetarian Resource Group for their extensive cookbook and reading list. One of my favorite general cookbooks is:

Ponichtera, Brenda. *Quick and Healthy Recipes and Ideas,* Volumes I and II (not completely vegetarian, but one of my favorites)

available from: 1519 Hermits Way
The Dalles, OR 97058
503-296-5859
503-296-1875

Books to help you adapt to your plant-based eating program

Havala, Suzanne. *The Vegetarian Food Guide and Nutrition Counter* (Berkeley Books, 1997).

Melina, Vesanto, Davis, Brenda, and Harrison, Victoria. *Becoming Vegetarian* (Book Publishing Company, 1996).

References

American Diabetes Association, Inc., and the American Dietetic Association. *Exchange Lists for Meal Planning.* 1995.

American Dietetic Association. "Fat Replacers: Position of the American Dietetic Association," *American Dietetic Association.* 1998; 98: 4.

American Dietetic Association. "USDA Rules Define 'Organic' Comments Sought on Labeling. Federal Update," *Journal of the American Dietetic Association.* 1998; 98: 4.

Armsey, Thomas, and Gary Green. "Nutrition Supplements: Science vs. Hype," *The Physician and Sportsmedicine.* 1997; 25: 6.

Avorn et al. "Reduction of Bacteria and Pyuria After Ingestion of Cranberry Juice," *Journal of the American Medical Association.* 1994; 271: 10.

Barker, Kenneth. *The New International Version Study Bible.* Ann Arbor, Michigan: Zondervan Corporation. 1985.

Bartas, Jeanne-Marie. "Vegan Menu Items at Fast Food and Family Style Restaurants—Part 1," *Vegetarian Journal,* Vegetarian Resource Group. 1997; pp. 16–19.

Benardot, Dan. *Sports Nutrition: A Guide for the Professional Working with Active People,* second edition. American Dietetic Association. 1993.

Bergeron, M. "Heat Cramps during Tennis: A Case Report." *International Journal of Sports Nutrition.* 1996; 6: pp. 62–68.

Berning, Jaqueline, and Suzanne Nelson. *Sports Nutrition for the 90's.* Gaithersburg, Maryland: Aspen, 1991.

———. *Nutrition for Sports and Exercise.* Gaithersburg, Maryland: Aspen, 1998.

Boyle, Marie, and Gail Zyla. *Personal Nutrition,* third edition. Minneapolis: West Publishing Company, 1996.

California Strawberry Commission, *Food for Thought: A Guide to Folic Acid.* (Pamphlet).

Carpenter, Ruth et al. *Questioning 40/30/30: A Guide to Understanding Sports Nutrition Advice.* (Brochure). The American Dietetic Association, The

American College of Sports Medicine, Women's Sports Foundation, and the Cooper Institute for Aerobics Research, p. 16.

Clarkson, Priscilla. "Nutritional Supplements for Weight Gain," *Sports Science Exchange*. Gatorade Sports Science Institute. 1998; 11: 1.

Clarkson, Priscilla, and Emily Haymes. "Exercise and Mineral Status of Athletes: Calcium, Magnesium, Phosphorus and Iron," *Medicine and Science in Sports and Exercise*. 1995; 27: 6: pp. 831–843.

Coleman, Ellen. "Nutrition Update: Fasting in Athletes," *Sports Medicine Digest*. 1985; 7: 4.

———. "Nutrition Update: Fat Loading Not Good for Endurance Exercise," *Sports Medicine Digest*. 1996; 18: 5.

———. "Alcohol and Performance," *Sports Medicine Digest*. 1997; 18: 10.

———. "Herbal Harm and Invisible Ephedrine," *Sports Medicine Digest*. 1997; 19: 5: pp. 57–58.

———. "A Dietary Twilight Zone," *Sports Medicine Digest*. 1997; 19: 9.

———. "Pyruvate Supplements: Fact vs. Fiction," *Sports Medicine Digest*. 1997; 19: 11.

Coyle, Edward. "Fat Metabolism During Exercise," *Sports Science Exchange*. Gatorade Sports Science Institute. 1995; 8: 6.

Craig, Winston. "Phytochemicals: Guardians of Our Health," *Issues in Vegetarian Dietetics*. 1996; 5: 3.

Davis, J. Mark. "Carbohydrates: Branched-Chain Amino Acids and Endurance: The Central Fatigue Hypothesis," *Sports Science Exchange*. Gatorade Sport Science Institute. 1995; 5.

DiPasquale, Mauro. *Amino Acids and Proteins for the Athlete: The Anabolic Edge*. Boca Raton: CRC Press. 1997.

Engelhardt, Martin, Georg Neumanne, Anneliese Berbalk, and Iris Reuter. "Creatine Supplementation in Endurance Sports," *Med Sci Sports Exerc*. 1998; 30: 7: pp. 1123–1129.

Frank, Laura. "The Chromium Chelator Question: Are Both Forms Equal?" *Scan's Pulse*. 1999; 18: p. 2.

Frankenfield, David, Eric Muth, and William Rowe. "The Harris-Benedict Studies of Human Basal Metabolism: History and Limitations," *J Am Diet Assoc*. 1998; 98: pp. 439–445.

Gatorade Sports Science Institute. "Caffeine and Endurance Performance," *Sports Science Exchange*. 1990; 3: 26.

Gisolfi, Carl. "Exercise, Intestinal Absorption and Rehydration," *Sports Science Exchange*. Gatorade Sports Science Institute. 1991; 4: 32.

Graham, Terry. "Caffeine and Exercise Performance," *Sports Science Exchange*. Gatorade Sports Science Institute. 1996; 9: 1.

Grandjean, Ann. "The Vegetarian Athlete," *The Physician and Sportsmedicine*. 1987: 15: 5.

Gutgesell, Margaret et al. "Reported Alcohol Use and Behavior in Long-Distance Runners," *Medicine and Science in Sports and Exercise*. 1996; 28: 8: pp. 1063–1070.

Hahn, Nancy. "Growing a Healthy Food System," *Journal of the American Dietetic Association.* 1997; 97: 9: pp. 949–950.

Hall, Nicholas. *Herbs, Hormones and the Mind.* Institute for CorText Research and Development. (Handout). Spring 1999.

Havakla, Suzanne. *The Vegetarian Food Guide and Nutrition Counter.* New York: Berkeley Books. 1997.

Heaney, Robert. "Calcium: How Your Diet Affects Requirements," *Vegetarian Nutrition & Health Newsletter.* Loma Linda University. 1998; 1: 3.

Horswill, Craig. "Effects of Bicarbonate, Citrate and Phosphate Loading on Performance," *International Journal of Sports Nutrition,* 1995; 5 (suppl).

Institute for Natural Resources. *Herbs, Vitamins and Neutraceuticals.* (Handout). 1999.

Ji, Li Li. "Exercise and Oxidative Stress: Role of the Cellular Antioxidant Systems," *Exercise and Sports Sciences Reviews.* 1995; 23.

Kannan, Srimathi. "Factors in Vegetarian Diets Influencing Iron and Zinc Bioavailablity," *Issues in Vegetarian Dietetics.* 1998; 7: 3.

Kapica, Cathy. "Phytochemicals: Getting Ready for the 21st Century," *DBC Dimensions Newsletter.* Winter 1996, p. 4.

Kim, Esther, Karen Schroeder, Robert Houser, and Johanna Dwyer. "Two Small Surveys, 25 Years Apart, Investigating Motivations of Dietary Choice in 2 Groups of Vegetarians in the Boston Area," *Journal of the American Dietetic Association.* 1999; 99: 5: pp. 598–601.

Klevay, Leslie. "Dietary Copper and Human Health," *Nutrition and the MD.* 1987; 13: 6.

Kolodinski, Elke. "Cycling with Caffeine: The Legal Performance Enhancer." *Bicyclist Magazine.* 1997.

Krause, Marie, and L. Kathleen Mahan. *Food, Nutrition and Diet Therapy,* seventh edition. Philadelphia: W.B. Saunders Company. 1984.

Larson, Enette. "Vegetarian Diet for Exercise, Athletic Training and Performing: An Update," *Issues in Vegetarian Nutrition.* 1997; VI: 3.

Lemon, Peter. "Do Athletes Need More Dietary Protein and Amino Acids?" *International Journal of Sports Nutrition.* 1995; 5 (suppl): pp. 39–61.

Linder, Maria. *Nutritional Biochemistry and Metabolism,* second edition. Norwalk, Connecticut: Appleton & Lange. 1991.

Lukaski, Henry. "Micronutrients (Magnesium, Zinc and Copper): Are Mineral Supplements Necessary for Athletes?" *The International Journal of Sports Nutrition.* 1995; 5 (suppl).

Matson, Larry, and Zung Vu Tran. "Effects of Sodium Bicarbonate Ingestion on Anaerobic Performance: A Meta-Analytic Review," *International Journal of Sports Nutrition.* 1993. 3: 1: pp. 2–28.

Maughan, Ronald. "Creatine Supplementation and Exercise Performance," *International Journal of Sports Nutrition.* 1995; 5: 2.

Murray, Bob. "Fluid Replacement: The American College of Sports Medicine Position Stand," *Sports Science Exchange.* Gatorade Sports Science Institute. 1996; 9: 4.

National Research Council. *Recommended Dietary Allowances,* tenth edition. Washington, DC: National Academy Press. 1989.

Nieman, David. "Vegetarian Dietary Practice and Endurance Performance," *Journal of Clinical Nutrition.* 1998; 48: pp. 754–761.

Nissen, Steven. "HMB Supplementation and Exercise," *Scan's Pulse.* Spring 1998; 17: 2.

Packer, Lester, and Vishwa Singh. "Nutrition and Exercise: Introduction and Overview," American Institute of Nutrition *Journal of Nutrition.* 1992; 122: pp. 758–759.

Pawlak, Laura. *A Perfect 10: Phyto "New-Trients" against Cancers.* Emeryville, California: Biomed General Corp. 1998.

Penn State Sports Medicine Newsletter. Water That Works Better. June 1994; 2: 10.

Rock, Cheryl, Robert Jacob, and Phyllis Bowen. "Update on the Biological Characteristics of the Antioxidant Micronutrients: Vitamin C, Vitamin E and the Caratenoids," *Journal of the American Dietetic Association.* 1996; 96; 7: pp. 693–702.

Rosenbloom, Chris. "Adrostenedione: Its Potential Safety Concerns," *Scan's Pulse.* 1999; 18: 2: pp. 4–6.

Running and Fitness News. "Androstenedione and Performance." 1998; 16: 12: p. 1.

Sherman, W. Michael, and Nicole Leenders. "Fat Loading: The Next Magic Bullet?" *International Journal of Sports Nutrition.* 1995; 5 (suppl): pp. 1–12.

Shils, Maurice, James Olson, and Moshe Shike. *Modern Nutrition in Health and Disease,* eighth edition. Philadelphia: Lea & Febiger. 1994.

Singh, Vishwa. "A Current Perspective on Nutrition and Exercise," *Journal of Nutrition.* American Institute of Nutrition. 1992; 122: pp. 760–765.

Sizer, Frances, and Eleanor Whitney. *Hamilton and Whitney's Nutrition Concepts and Controversies,* sixth edition. Minneapolis/St. Paul: West Publishing Company. 1994.

Smolin, Lori, and Mary Grosvenor. *Nutrition Science and Applications,* second edition. Fort Worth: Saunders Publishing. 1997.

Snape, William. "Nutrients and Gastric Emptying," *Nutrition and the MD.* 1996; 12: 11.

Sports, Cardiovascular and Wellness Nutritionists. "Ergogenic Aids: Reported Facts and Claims," *Scan's Pulse.* 1998; (suppl).

Strailey, Jennifer. "The Neutraceutical Revolution," *The Gourmet Retailer Magazine.* 1997; pp. 153–157.

Thompson, Janice. "Predicted and Measured Resting Metabolic Rate of Male and Female Endurance Athletes," *Journal of the American Dietetic Association.* 1996; 96: 1.

Tinley, Scott. "You Are What You Eat." *Triathlon Magazine.* 1997.

Traegar James. *The Food Chronology.* New York: Holt and Company. 1995.

Tufts Diet and Nutrition Newsletter. "Clearing Up Common Misconceptions about Vegetarianism." 1998; 16: 2: pp. 4–5.

Tyler, Varro. *The Honest Herbal.* New York: Haworth Press, Inc. 1993.

Ulene, Art. *Fat and Cholesterol in Your Food.* Avery Publishing Group. 1995.

United States Olympic Committee. *SportsMed 2000 Information Packet.* Colorado Springs, Colorado.

Vegetarian Diets. "Position of the American Dietetic Association." 1997; 97: 11, pp. 1317–1321.

Vegetarian Times Magazine. "Food Fight." April 1998; pp. 73–80.

Volek, Jeff. Creatine Monohydrate: "Is It a Performance Enhancer?" *Scan Pulse.* Sports, Cardiovascular and Wellness Nutritionists, Fall 1996.

Vyhmeister, Irma. "Advantages of Vegetarian Diets," *Nutrition and the MD.* 1984; 10: 6.

———. "Vegetarian Diets—Issues and Concerns," *Nutrition and the MD.* 1984; 10: 5.

Wagner, Dale. "Hyperhydrating with Glycerol: Implications for Athletic Performance." *Journal of the American Dietetic Association.* 1999; 99: pp. 207–212.

Weinsier, Roland. "Branched-Chain Amino Acids in Stressed Surgical Patients," *Nutrition and the MD.* 1985; 11: 9.

White, Randall, Jennifer Seymour, and Erica Frank. "Vegetarianism among U.S. Women Physicians," *Journal of the American Dietetic Association.* 1999; 99: 5: pp. 595–598.

Wilcox, Anthony. "Caffeine and Endurance Performance," *Sports Science Exchange.* Gatorade Sports Science Institute. 1990; 3: 26.

Williams, Clyde, and Ceri Nicholas. "Nutrition Needs for Team Sport," *Sports Science Exchange.* Gatorade Sports Science Institute. 1998; 11: 3.

Williams, Melvin. *The Competitive Edge at Any Price: The Use of Ergogenic Aids Among Athletes.* SCAN Symposium. Houston Texas. 1988.

———. "Bicarbonate Loading," *Sports Science Exchange.* Gatorade Sports Science Institute. 1992; 4: 36.

Williams, Paul. "Interactive Effects of Exercise, Alcohol and Vegetarian Diet on Coronary Artery Disease Risk Factors in 9,242 Runners: The National Runners' Health Study," *American Journal of Clinical Nutrition.* 1997; 66: 1197–1206.

Wilson, Peter. "Importance of Zinc in Human Nutrition," *Nutrition and the MD.* 1994; 10: 2.

Wolinsky, Ira, and Judy Driskell. *Sports Nutrition: Vitamins and Trace Elements.* Boca Raton: CRC Press. 1997.

Zaloga, Gary. *Biological Effects of Food Components: Modulation of Immunity.* (Handout). American Dietetic Association Annual Meeting. October 1998.

Index